Mediterranean Meals to Your Health

10-Day Detox to Reset Your Metabolism, Reach Your Ideal Weight
& Start Craving Healthy Foods

ISBN: **978-1511836340**

The information in this book is provided to describe the health benefits of the Mediterranean diet. However, any decision involving the treatment of an illness should be made only after consulting the physician of your choice.

Neither this nor any other book can guarantee complete absence of disease nor substitute for professional medical care or treatment.

The information contained in this book is not intended to serve as a replacement for professional medical advice. Any use of the information in this book is at the reader's discretion.

The authors specifically disclaim any and all liability arising directly or indirectly from the use or application of any information contained in this ebook. A health care professional should be consulted regarding your specific situation.

Table of Contents

Introduction:

For most people, the word diet brings to mind deprivation and misery. This is because most of the diet bandwagons people get onto are restrictive, unhealthy, not feasible as long-term lifestyles, and offer no way to keep the weight off after it's gone. To get the weight off and keep it off while getting and staying healthy, you need to skip the fad diets and adopt a new, healthier lifestyle. I'm here to show you how.

What to Expect from Reading this Book

By the time you finish this book, you will have learned:

- Why it's so important to listen to your body and how to do so,
- How to control your impulses and eat the right things,
- Why drastically controlling your intake of fat, carbs, cholesterol, or anything else will actually backfire, and
- How to prepare balanced meals that provide all the nutrients you need,

Everyone knows that losing weight is a simple matter of burning more calories than you consume, but this is an oversimplified formula. Many people take this to mean that losing weight means eating less. However, when faced with severe calorie restriction, the body assumes you are in a famine situation and responds by slowing metabolism and conserving calories rather than burning them.

The real key to losing weight has nothing to do with counting calories, but about eating a nutritious and balanced diet. By the time you finish reading this book, you'll know exactly what that looks like and how to do it.

It's no secret that a Mediterranean-style diet can help you reach your ideal weight, flatten your belly and improve your overall health in just 7 days.

And starting from today you can achieve more in less time by overeating the foods you love!

YES! The new meal planner creates personalized meal plans to achieve your goals quickly. All plans fit perfectly to your tastes, budget, skills and lifestyle.

Then just go grocery shopping, follow the meal plan with recipes, and reach your health goals without even trying. Never think about what you should eat ever again.

You can choose your own eating style, including Mediterranean, low carb, gluten-free, vegan, diabetic, and many more via the extensive options menu.

You can print out menus, recipes and shopping lists, and we'll make sure you have plenty of variety so you'll never get bored.

If you need to lose weight, you'll melt those extra pounds. If you don't need to lose, you'll get a custom plan to improve your health, boost your energy level and feel good all over.

Simply Sit, Relax and Enjoy the Foods You Love...We'll Take Care of All That Comes with It!

Get it here → http://www.mediterraneanbook.com/28day/

The Basic Principles of the Meals to Your Health Diet

A diet consisting of processed foods devoid of actual nutrition, combined with a sedentary lifestyle, is a major cause of death and disease in the world today.

There are many reasons why people decide they want to lose weight. They know losing weight lowers risk of disease, increases confidence, and just all around helps people feel better and be healthier. A slender and attractive appearance is just icing on the cake of a healthy lifestyle.

The MEALS TO YOUR HEALTH diet isn't just a diet that is followed for a few weeks or months, it's a lifestyle change that will help you lose weight, keep it off, and improve your overall health.

Eliminating processed foods and replacing them with high quality, nutritious, natural food in reasonable portions is the main premise behind the MEALS TO YOUR HEALTH diet. Making small, gradual changes will lead you to a healthy lifestyle that will help you achieve the weight you want.

Add moderate exercise to healthy eating, and you will be able to burn more calories every day, helping you to lose weight faster.

How to Start Easily

Many fad diets and gimmicks promise rapid weight loss, and it's common to be tempted to give them a try. The problem is that even when they work, it's also common for the weight to come right back.

Losing weight gradually, at a rate of a pound or two per week, is a healthier and more sustainable approach. Losing weight gradually, over a period of six months or even a year, is easier to both achieve and maintain than losing the same amount in a month or two.

It's not necessary to diet, to deprive yourself, or to spend money on diet pills or diet foods. All you need to do is eat a variety of nutritious foods in reasonable portions.

At this point, it's normal to wonder how you're going to change your current dietary habits.

Unhealthy eating habits don't happen overnight, they usually build over many years, even decades. When you think about changing these deep seated patterns, it can seem impossible, especially if you are trying to convince your spouse and the rest of your family to adopt healthier habits as well.

Changing your habits doesn't have to be as hard as it seems, especially if you shift your lifestyle gradually, rather than eliminating all of your favorites at once.

When you gradually replace junk foods with healthier options, it gives you a chance to adjust gradually and find new foods that you can enjoy without feeling deprived. Sudden change can be a huge shock to the system, while gradual change leads to a healthy lifestyle in a way that is much easier to maintain long term.

The best way to set a foundation for healthy change is to ensure you have healthy foods in your refrigerator and pantry. Rather than throwing everything out and restocking from scratch, it's much easier to replace items with healthier version whenever you shop to replace items you've run out of.

Getting Results Fast

It's perfectly normal to want to see results as soon as you start changing the way you eat. Overcoming a lifetime of bad habits is a lot of work, and it can be discouraging to do all that and not notice any change in how you feel.

Rest assured, if you stick with your healthier lifestyle, eating nutritious foods and exercising regularly, you'll notice a difference within a month.

With gradual and consistent changes, balanced meals, and moderate exercise, weight loss of seven pounds in the first month is perfectly doable. Keep going, and you can easily drop and additional seven pounds in the second month, and the gains (or losses, rather!) keep adding up.

Not only will you lose weight, you'll start looking and feeling better, and find yourself with more energy. All of these will give you the motivation to keep going with your new, healthy lifestyle.

Staying Motivated

Losing weight isn't easy, keeping it off is even harder. It's important to find ways to keep yourself focused on the long term benefits so you don't slip back into old habits. Here are some of our favorite ways to stay motivated:

Focus on the benefits - There are lots of ways to motivate yourself, but one of the best is to focus on the benefits directly related to your changes, including:

Cholesterol - Eating healthier and losing weight will lower your cholesterol and with it, your risk of cardiovascular disease.

Diabetes - According to the Centers for Disease Control, nearly ten percent of the US adult population has Type II diabetes. Losing just ten pounds of excess weight can lower your risk.

High blood pressure - Losing weight and exercising regularly can help you maintain a healthy blood pressure.

Cancer - Eating a nutritious diet reduces your risk of many types of cancer.

Don't let one bad day thwart your efforts. Sooner or later, you're going to have one of those days where you just need to indulge. Plan ahead for days like this, treat yourself, then get back on track. Tomorrow is another day, and another opportunity to do better. The longer you do this, the easier it gets.

Focus on positives - Don't underestimate how much your attitude will influence your efforts. Keep your goal in sight, but keep your focus on how much you've already accomplished, and don't worry about how much farther you have to go.

Remember your reasons for changing - You're not going through all of this for nothing, you have reasons for losing weight. When you keep these in mind, it will be less stressful to change your lifestyle than to keep the weight.

Be prepared for challenging situations - Holidays and other special occasions can pose particular temptations. It can be tempting to skip meals in order to cut down on calories in preparation, but this can lead to over indulging. It is also helpful to exercise before or after the event. Exercise before to curb your appetite, and after to burn calories.

Avoid people who would undermine your efforts, but don't rely on others to keep you on track. This is your journey and it's up to you to keep yourself going.

Be patient - you're in a marathon, not a sprint.

Change it up - When you find yourself on a plateau, find a new exercise or physical activity.

Watch your portion sizes - It's easy to eat more than you think you are.

Be realistic - A pound or two a week is a healthy rate of weight loss. More than that, and you start losing muscle and doing yourself more harm than good.

Reward yourself - Before you even get started, decide on some meaningful rewards to help keep you going. Some ideas include:

Movie or play

Vacation, cruise, or day trip

New outfit, book, or CD

Concert

Trip to the spa

New cookware

New gadget

The sky's the limit!

Overeating is most often the result of stress, feeling deprived, or other emotion, not actual hunger.

Many diets require you to eliminate many favorite comfort foods and leave you feeling deprived. When you encounter stressful situations, it can be tempting to indulge. The problem doesn't come when you enjoy your favorite foods, the problem comes when you binge because you've been so good for so long.

The good news is, you can protect yourself from this eventuality by incorporating small amounts of your favorite foods on occasion. This will keep you from feeling deprived.

Women most frequently report craving chocolate, while men more frequently crave meat and salty snacks. The one thing nearly all of the commonly craved foods have in common is caloric density, so it's unsurprising that overweight people often report strong cravings.

That said, there's not scientific evidence to back the idea that avoiding certain foods intensifies cravings for those foods. In fact, the reverse is often true. While you might seem to want a food more when you first start avoiding it, those cravings should subside in time.

Overcoming Cravings

It's well known that stress causes both physical and mental strain and can interfere with your ability to make good decisions. Learning to manage your stress levels now can help you avoid stick to your plan.

Binge eating is a disorder where a person consumes unusually large amounts of food. Here are some strategies to overcoming binge eating:

- Avoid baking and cooking deserts and other tempting foods

- Exercise

- Keep a food diary and note down what you eat and how much

- Clear your cupboards and fridge of junk food

- Eat regular 3 meals per day and healthy snacks in between

- Don't eat in front of the T.V.

- Avoid the temptation – the urge to eat may eventually pass

Here are some more tips to keep you away from binge eating:

- Stay away from tempting foods that you would normally like to indulge on

- Avoid taking second helpings from the buffet table

- Turn up late and leave early at the table.

- Help out with table setting or start cleaning up the kitchen as soon as you have eaten

Eating at "Bad Times": Depression and binge eating are connected to each other. When we find ourselves in any sort of stressful situations, we use food as a way to cope with it. For example, if a person has a breakup, he/she is more likely to turn to chocolate or ice-cream. You can avoid overeating when you are feeling down by:

- Take extra care of yourself

- Exercise is not only good for a healthy lifestyle, but it also helps in reducing stress and lifting depression. By exercising regularly, you will feel less urge to eat especially at emotional times

- Do something special for yourself when you are down. Go to the parlor, get a makeover, buy some new clothes, go to the movies or games to take your mind off the stressful situation

- Get support from friends or a binge support group

Sometimes people overeat when they have low self-esteem. Many times, we find ourselves in situations where someone says something bad about you or you make an embarrassing mistake in front of your colleagues. These situations make us unhappy and on a bad day, the food seems like our only friend.

Binge eating makes the feelings of stress; anxiety, depression, and loneliness evaporate into the air. But this is only temporary. To find a permanent cure, we have to overcome the feelings of stress. This can be resolved by handling stress through meditation, exercise, practicing simple breathing exercises, or using other types of relaxation strategies.

Irregular eating or skipping meals will also trigger your food cravings and the urge to overeat. Eat regular meals and make proper nutrition choices. Always eat a balanced diet which has a variety of foods from all food groups. Make sure that you are getting sufficient vitamins and minerals from your diet. Making the right food choices will help you cope with overeating and manage stress.

Boredom:

Many times, people eat to fight boredom. We all like to snack while watching TV or surfing the internet. When we are doing two activities at one time, we tend to eat large quantities of food.

Instead of eating when you are bored, distract yourself from the boredom. Try going for a walk on commercial breaks or read a book. You can also work on a craft like knitting while watching TV.

If you are overeating when you don't want to:

- Keep healthy foods in your cupboard and freezer

- Ask yourself why you overate when you didn't want to. Were you feeling low? How can you change your emotional behavior?

- Don't dwell on it. That will make you unhappy. You can try again the next day

- Try decreasing your food intake each day

- Exercise

- Find another activity to do for the next time you feel the urge to overeat

- If you find yourself in the same stressful situation regularly, change your routine

Chocolate Craving Solutions

If you have chocolate cravings, here are some tips to replace the chocolate with low-calorie food items:

- Cocoa powder can be used as a substitute for chocolate. You can sprinkle it on coffee or yogurt.

- Dark chocolate can also help satisfy your chocolate cravings in few bites

- Eat a small chocolate biscuit instead of a chocolate bar to cope with your chocolate cravings

How to Avoid Hunger Attacks

The biggest obstacle for many people trying to lead a healthier lifestyle is between meal hunger that can lead to an urge to snack.

When hunger strikes and the next meal is hours away, it can be easy to give in to an impulse to grab the first thing that looks like it will quell the craving. This is often something with lots of calories, but little or no nutritional value, such as chips or a candy bar.

The best way to avoid hunger pangs is to consume your calories in well space meals throughout the day and snacking on fruit and other nutritious, low calorie foods in between. By eating this way, you'll be able to cut your calorie intake without feeling hungry.

The trick is to make breakfast your largest and most substantial meal of the day, eat a moderate lunch, and make dinner your smallest meal. The large breakfast will give you plenty of energy to get you through the day and ramp up your metabolism for the day. A small dinner will minimize the number of calories you consume shortly before bed, when your metabolism is a bit slower.

Feel Full on Fewer Calories

Fad diets typically don't work for the simple fact that they often leave you feeling hungry. The best way to consume fewer calories is to consume them in the form of high nutrition foods that will actually help you feel full. It's not only unnecessary to starve yourself, it's counterproductive.

A good way to reduce your calorie intake without even notice is to eat slowly and chew thoroughly. Research has found that food is much less satisfying when it is consumed via feeding tube than it is when eaten normally.

This would suggest that the sensory experience of eating, including the feel, taste, and smell of the food are important to communicating information to the brain about the amount of calories consumed.

It would also suggest that the more thoroughly you chew your food, the more quickly your body will release hormones associated with satiety, the faster you will feel full, and the fewer calories you will consume.

Unprocessed and minimally processed foods are lower in calories and higher in fiber and nutrition than most of the highly processed foods that are such a big part of the modern diet.

Best Foods to Eat

- High in water
- High in fiber
- Low in calorie density
- Low in fat
- No added sugar

GO! foods are generally those with a high water content. Gluten-free grains such as oatmeal, barley, quinoa, brown rice, and gluten-free pasta are better than foods like bread or crackers. That's not to say you should eliminate bread or crackers, but they should be eaten in moderation.

Other GO! foods include: fresh fruits and vegetables, cooked gluten-free whole grains, and lean protein. These foods are packed with nutrition and high in a variety of vitamins and minerals.

Use Portion Control!

- Protein, salmon, tuna, swordfish
- Dried fruit, jams
- Desserts, cheesecake, apple pie, ice cream

These foods are generally fairly nutritious, but they are much higher in calories and generally contain less nutrition and are less satisfying than GO! foods. Enjoy these foods in moderation.

Go Very Easy on These

- Refined carbs, muffins, cookies, fat-free pretzels
- Refined carbs, bread sticks, dry cereals, crackers
- Cheese, cheddar cheese, Swiss, Brie, etc.
- Regular treats, refined potato chips, cookies, candy, brownies, fudge, regular crackers.
- High-fat products, chocolate candy, nuts &seeds
- High-fat products, bacon, margarine, butter, mayo
- Fats and oils, lard, vegetable oil, shortening

These foods are less satisfying, less nutritious, and more calorie dense than the other categories. You don't have to eliminate these foods, but enjoy them as an occasional treat.

Did you know that it's really easy to figure out calorie density just by looking at the label? Compare the number of grams in a serving to the number of calories. If there are fewer calories than grams, the food has low caloric density.

Vinegar Prevents Hunger Attacks

A recent study conducted by Carol Johnston, PhD, RD at Arizona State University found vinegar to be highly effective at moderating the increase in blood sugar from consuming foods that are high in carbohydrates.

Johnston provided a meal that was high in carbohydrates to subjects who had both normal and elevated blood sugar levels. Before the meal, subjects were given drinks containing either a placebo or 2 tablespoons of vinegar, and each subject's blood sugar levels were measured before and after the meal.

In subjects with prediabetes or impaired glucose tolerance, the increase in blood sugar levels was 34% less than similar individuals who had been given the placebo. In individuals with type 2 diabetes and those with normal blood sugar showed an increase in blood sugar 20% lower in the vinegar group than in the placebo group.

It seems that the acetic acid in the vinegar inhibits the enzyme responsible for digesting starch, slowing its absorption. Blood sugar levels spike when starch is broken down and absorbed rapidly.

Eating a big salad with vinegar based dressing before lunch and dinner should enhance weight loss both by decreasing overall calorie intake and slowing digestion of starches from potatoes and other high-GI foods. Doing this can help prevent blood sugar spikes, especially in diabetic individuals, as well as reducing nutritional stress on beta cells.

How to Portion Control

Changing your lifestyle may seem daunting, but it doesn't have to be difficult. You can make changes. All you need to do is embrace health and let excitement get you through the initial difficulty and you'll be fine.

One of the most important factors in eating healthier and losing weight is portion control. Even nutritious food can hamper your weight loss efforts when you eat too much.

Portion control is vital, but the idea of counting calories and carefully measuring portions at every meal can be intimidating.

Consuming large portions both at home and when eating out is one of the biggest obstacles encountered today. Disproportionately large servings of food have become normal, but there are some visual tricks you can use to keep your servings reasonable without spending time weighing or measuring.

One simple technique is to mentally divide your plate into sections.

Half the plate is allotted to fruits and vegetables. The other half is then divided in half, so that a quarter of the plate is for protein and the last quarter to gluten-free grain. Master this method, and you'll have no trouble managing your portions visually.

Be cautious with the following 7 foods:

1. Beverages – Beverages are a major source of refined and added sugar in most people's diets, especially when you consider the amount most people drink in a day. The common rule of thumb is eight 8-oz glasses (or 64 oz) of

water per day. Every time you substitute juice, soda, sports drinks, or other beverages for water, you're adding sugar and empty calories that do not actually contribute to satiety. Drink plenty of pure water, and you'll be ahead of the game.

2. Chips and crackers – These foods are so convenient to grab and munch as you go about your day. However, these foods are very calorie dense, with serving sizes usually about an ounce. Eating these foods while doing other things can quickly lead to mindless overeating. Keep fruits and veggies on hand for healthy, low calorie grab and go snacks.

3. Baked goods – You may be shocked at how many calories are in a seemingly normal sized cookie or cake from a bakery. A single serving of an item in a bakery may easily be 500 calories or more. Compare this to an 80 calorie apple.

4. Fried food – A good way to double the calorie content of food is to fry it. Go with foods that are grilled, baked, roasted, steamed, or raw.

5. Pizza – Pizza is an easy food to overdo, often taking two or three times as much as you should eat to get full. When you indulge, start with a large salad and omit the cheese, or at least go easy on it.

6. Salad – Wait, what? Salad is good for you, isn't it? It is, until you add a bunch of creamy dressing and high-fat toppings such as bacon and croutons. Go ahead and eat as much salad as you care to, but leave off the high fat toppings and swap the creamy dressing for one that is vinegar based.

7. Meat – Many cuts are significantly more than a 3 oz. serving. Limit your serving of chicken or fish to a quarter of your plate. Red meat should only be eaten occasionally.

The biggest key to making better choices about what you eat is awareness. Many people have just a couple of foods that present obstacles when it comes to overindulging. It may be potato chips or crackers, cookies or snack cakes, or you may be fine at home, but have trouble when you eat out. The next couple of chapters will show you how to deal with these problems.

Breakfast Ideas

Breakfast is a great way to jumpstart your metabolism for the day with essential nutrients and fiber for energy throughout the day. Starting the day with a healthy breakfast is a great way to cut overall calories for the day.

These foods are great for breakfast:

- Gluten-free cereals,
- Fresh fruit,
- Fresh vegetables,
- Egg whites,
- Nuts or nut butters

Cereals, fruits, and vegetables are great sources of fiber, while protein helps you feel full longer. As important as breakfast is, many people frequently skip it, either because they don't have time or aren't hungry in the mornings.

Here are some ways to find time:

- Prepare something the night before. Better yet, spend a couple of hours over the weekend putting together breakfast foods for the week.

- Stock healthy, quick, and easy breakfast items on hand.
- Get up a few minutes earlier.

Here are some ways to get hungry in the morning:

- Get up a little earlier to give yourself a little more time to get hungry.
- Go for an early morning walk or get some other exercise to work up an appetite.
- Plan a breakfast that you can take with you, such as a breakfast burrito or smoothie.
- If it's feasible at your job, eat breakfast at work, either at your desk or during a morning break.

Quick, Easy, Delicious, and Nutritious Breakfast Ideas

- Yogurt with fruit, and whole-grain toast or topped with whole-grain cereal,
- Egg-white sandwich with fruit and almond or other non-dairy milk,
- Cereal made from gluten-free whole grains with non-dairy milk and fruit,
- English muffin with nut butter spread and a piece of fruit,
- Oatmeal topped with raisins and a glass of non-dairy milk,
- Muffins made from gluten-free whole grains (these are good for making ahead and freezing),
- Pancakes or waffles topped with fruit compote (another good make ahead option),
- Breakfast burritos filled with scrambled egg whites, fresh veggies, salsa, and beans.

What's not to love about salad? Salads are delicious and packed with fiber and nutrition. If you are trying to lose weight, eating a daily salad can get you to your goal even faster.

Research has shown that people who eat salad with low-fat dressing and toppings before a meal consume fewer calories for the meal than those who did not. Another study found that acetic acid found in vinegar may help you feel more satisfied after eating.

More research may be needed to determine all of the benefits of eating salad regularly, but existing research indicates that eating a salad with nutritious toppings is a great idea. Be sure to use a vinegar based dressing, as vinegar is naturally fat-free, low sodium, and packed with flavor.

Best Salad Toppings

Fresh vegetables and fruit, dried tomatoes, nuts and seeds, lemon zest, and peppers are all great options for adding flavor and texture and increasing the nutritional value of the salad. Vinegar or lemon juice are good dressing options if you are trying to lose weight.

Worst Salad Toppings

Cheese, creamy dressings, crouton, and bacon bits are all high in fat, calories, and sodium. Go easy on these toppings, or omit them entirely.

Save Time

- Make a large salad without the dressing. This way you can munch on the same salad for a few days.

- Add grilled chicken or fish to a salad for an easy, healthy entrée.
- Scoop some salad into a pita to eat on the go.

Try some of the following flavorful vinegars with your salad: white, red, or rice wine vinegar, balsamic vinegar, cider vinegar, or raspberry vinegar. If you're feeling adventurous, try making your own flavored vinegars with herbs, spices, or fruit.

Snack Smart

Research has shown that spreading out calories across three small meals rather than eating the same number of calories in one large meal can help you consume fewer at your next meal. The reason for this is that, when you wait too long to eat, you get hungrier and are more likely to overeat. Instead of eating three large meals, try consuming 5 or 6 smaller meals at regular intervals. Not only will this prevent you from getting hungry enough to overeat, it will keep your metabolism burning calories at a more consistent rate through the day.

Be careful when eating bagged snacks like crackers and chips, as it can be hard to gauge how much you're eating. Look for 100 calorie snack packs, or get some snack size containers and portion out your snacks yourself. Portioning snacks yourself is quite a bit less expensive than buying the individual sized packages.

If you're going to portion out snacks yourself, it's a good idea to do it all at once when you get home from the store. This way you don't have big bags or boxes of food in the cabinet to grab and eat mindlessly. It also makes it easy to grabs snacks to eat on the go. You can also cut up fresh fruit or veggies to put in a baggie or container to grab on the run as well.

However you plan your snack portions, be sure you are actually hungry when you eat and not bored, anxious, or experience any other negative emotions. A good way to determine this is to ask yourself if you're hungry enough to eat broccoli. If you are, you're hungry. If not, odds are you're wanting to eat for other reasons.

Super Snacks

The food industry would have you believe that snacks aren't meant to be as nutritious as mealtime foods. Don't fall for it. Steer clear of packaged snack foods and think of your snacks as mini-meals.

- Soup – When we're talking salad dressing you want to avoid creamy, but the opposite is true for soup. Creamy soups are more filling than others, but since soup is usually eaten hot, it's not eaten quickly, so you are less likely to overdo.
- Yogurt – Fat-free or lowfat yogurt is packed with calcium and protein. Buy plain yogurt and add your own fruit. Be sure to read the label to avoid added sugar.
- Leftovers – After a nutritious dinner, pack your leftovers in the fridge for later snacking. It doesn't get much easier than this.
- Half a sandwich – Put some sandwich ingredients on a slice of whole grain bread or a pita.
- Baked potato or baked sweet potato – Put one in a steamer bag in the microwave for 4-5 minutes.
- Oatmeal – Not just for breakfast anymore. Add some cinnamon or nutmeg and a handful of dried fruit.
- Peanut butter and crackers – Use brown rice crackers and a tablespoon of peanut butter, top with a slice of fresh fruit.
- Bunny bag – Put some carrot sticks, cucumber slices,

sliced bell pepper, orange wedges, apple slices, raw cauliflower, or raw broccoli together in a zip lock bag or air tight container. The orange wedges will help keep the apple slices from turning brown.

- Smoothie – Pour some soy, almond, or rice milk into a blender, add some fruit and blend to make a satisfyingly delicious drink similar to a milkshake.
- Vegetable juice – This is a great way to get your vegetables in.
- Wrap – Put some turkey or chicken in a whole-grain tortilla with some lettuce leaves and diced tomato.
- Parfait – Layer fruit, grain, and low fat or nonfat yogurt in a cup.

Don't Drink Your Calories!

Nearly half of all sugar in the modern diet is consumed in liquid form. It's easy to underestimate how many calories you're consuming in drinks other than water.

Coffee contains almost no calories itself, but adding cream and sugar can increase the calorie content significantly. Each teaspoon of creamer or tablespoon of sugar adds an additional 45 calories each. Adding one of each adds 90 calories to a cup of coffee. Drinking just one cup per day of coffee with one teaspoon of creamer and a tablespoon of sugar adds an additional 32,850 calories over the course of a year.

According to a study conducted at Purdue University and published in the International Journal of Obesity, liquid calories such as those found in soda, sports drinks, or sweet tea don't register as food in terms of satiety, though they certainly count when it comes to trying to lose weight.

Participants ate 450 calories worth of jelly beans daily for a four week period, and drink 450 calories worth of soda daily for a second four week period. During the period when participants ate the jelly beans, they ate about 450 fewer calories worth of other foods. During the period when they drank the soda, they did not compensate for the soda and ended up consuming 450 more calories than they did before.

The point of this isn't that you should only ever drink water, black coffee and unsweetened tea, simply try to drink more of these no calorie beverages and be aware of how many calories you're consuming.

You should also be aware of how large that drink cup really is. Go to Burger King and order a king-size soda, and you'll be consuming 35 ounces, more than a quart.

Finally, many places offer unlimited refills, which can lead to drinking even more than intended without you really even thinking about it.

Lower Your Fat Intake

Fat is an important part of your diet, but consuming too much fat, or the wrong kinds, are known to contribute to many common modern diseases.

What Fat Does

- Store calories to provide energy
- Insulate the body
- Absorb, store, and transport certain nutrients
- Promote healthy skin and hair
- Comprises 60% of the brain

While some nutrients, such as certain vitamins, can be synthesized in the body, this is not true of essential fatty acids, they must come from the diet. This does not mean that a high fat diet is healthy, however, moderation is key.

Tricks to Ensure You get the Right Amount of the Right Kinds of Fat

- Calcium fortified, non-dairy milk contains 5 fewer grams of saturated fat than whole milk.
- Use less oil
    - When using oil in a recipe, measure it carefully,
    - In many recipes, you can use half the oil called for,
    - When greasing a pan or cookie sheet, use a spray can or mister to distribute evenly with the least amount possible,
    - Substitute broth for flavoring and sautéing. Broth is especially delicious in pastas and vegetables.
- Opt for lean cuts of meat and remove excess fat. Remove skin from poultry. White meat chicken or turkey is leaner than most cuts of red meat. Ground white meat turkey is a good substitute for hamburger, but be sure it's all white meat, ground turkey that contains dark meat or skin can be as high in fat as hamburger.
- Skip frying and go with low-fat methods of cooking such as baking, grilling, roasting, steaming, or poaching.
- Substitute two egg whites or a tablespoon of ground flax seed mixed with three tablespoons of water for a whole egg.
- Opt for oil and vinegar or lemon juice for salads. If you absolutely must have creamy ranch or blue cheese, have it on the side and dip your fork in the dressing before taking a bite of salad.

- At a restaurant, choose lower fat items in smaller portions. Request sauces on the side and ask if lower fat cooking methods are possible.

Foods List

Food	Tips	Eat	The Good	The Bad
Fruits:				
Apples ✓	Avoid pesticides by going organic	OK	High in fiber and antioxidants	
Apricots		OK	Plenty of antioxidants	
Avocado ✓		OK	Healthy fat source and high in B vitamins.	
Banana ✓		OK	High in fiber and prebiotics, helpful in lowering blood pressure.	
Blueberries ✓	Buy local and in season. Wash before eating and eat within 2-3 days. Good on salad.	OK	Antioxidant and protects the brain.	
Cantaloupe ✓		Eat moderately	Antioxidant and helps reduce Blood Pressure	
Cherries	Avoid ✓ pesticides by going organic	Eat moderately	Anti-inflammatory, good source of folic acid and antioxidants	
Grapes ✓	Buy local and in season. Wash before eating and eat within 2-3 days. Good on salad. Avoid pesticides by going organic.	OK	Anti-inflammatory, high in resveratrol and other antioxidants, protects the brain.	
Kiwi ✓		Eat moderately	High in antioxidants	

Food	Tips	Eat	The Good	The Bad
Oranges (Lemons, Lime, Grapefruit, Citrus, Tangerine) ✓	Buy local and in season. Wash before eating and eat within 2-3 days. Good on salad. Avoid pesticides by going organic.	OK	Antioxidant, anti-inflammatory, lowers blood pressure and cholesterol.	
Peaches	Buy local and in season. Wash before eating and eat within 2-3 days. Good on salad. Avoid pesticides by going organic.	OK	Antioxidant, anti-inflammatory, lowers cholesterol.	
Peaches, Canned in Syrup		OK	Watch for the sugar content. They may not maintain 100% of their nutrients.	
Pears ✓	Avoid pesticides by going organic.	OK		
Pear, canned in pear juice ✓		OK	Look on the label for the sugar content. Canning destroys some nutrients	
Pineapple ✓		Eat mode rately	Antioxidant	
Pomegranate		OK	Anti Inflammatory, Antioxidant	
Prunes		Eat mode rately		
Strawberries ✓	Avoid pesticides by going organic.	OK	Antioxidant, high in Calcium and Iron	

Food	Tips	Eat	The Good	The Bad
Watermelon ✓	Buy local and in season. Wash before eating and eat within 2-3 days. Good on salad.	OK	High in lycopene and other antioxidants, good for the heart.	
Dried Fruit:				
Dried Apples		Eat mode rately	High in Fiber and Antioxidants	Check the label for sugar and calories
Dried Apricots		Eat mode rately	High in Fiber and Antioxidants	Check the label for sugar and calories
Dried Dates		Eat mode rately		
Dried Figs		Eat mode rately	High in calcium and antioxidants, lowers blood pressure.	Check the label for sugar and calories
Dried Prunes		Eat mode rately	High in Fiber and Antioxidants	Check the label for sugar and calories
Raisins	Sweet, can use in place of sugar	Eat mode rately	Antioxidant and good source of Iron	Check the label for sugar and calories
Grains:				
Barley ✓	Simmer 10-12 min.	OK	Revs up metabolism, lowers cholesterol, feeds beneficial gut bacteria, high in antioxidants.	
Basmati ✓ Rice		OK		

Food	Tips	Eat	The Good	The Bad
Breakfast Cereals	Avoid sweetened cereals	Eat moderately		Watch for added sugar.
Brown Rice ✓	No need to rinse, Cook in the oven for about an hour.	OK	High in fiber and antioxidants, good source of iron lowers cholesterol and inflammation, revs up metabolism.	
Buckwheat	Good in soups.	OK		
Bulgur		Eat moderately		
Corn ✓		OK		High glycemic index with low nutritional value, One of the most common GMO.
Couscous ✓		OK		
Millet	Good in cakes, biscuits or soups.	OK	Eases acid reflux, hHigh in antioxidant, revs up Metabolism and lowers cholesterol	
Muesli		Eat moderately	Good source of Fiber	Watch sugar content
Oatmeal	Perfect breakfast food. Steel cut is best, avoid instant.	OK	Good source of calcium and antioxidants, revs metabolism, lower cholesterol and blood pressure.	

Food	Tips	Eat mode rately	The Good	The Bad
Pasta	Cook "al dente" (slightly firm) to make improve satiety. ✓	Eat mode rately	Antioxidant, revs up Metabolism	Contains gluten
Quinoa ✓	Simmer over medium low 15 min.	OK	Antioxidant, revs up Metabolism, good source of protein	
Brown Rice Pasta ✓		OK		
Spelt	Good in soups or to make bread.	OK	Antioxidant, revs up Metabolism, Lowers cholesterol	
White Rice	Eat less than once a week ?	NO		High glycemic index.
Whole Wheat Pasta ✓	Cook "al dente" (slightly firm) to make improve satiety.	OK	Antioxidant, revs up Metabolism, Lowers cholesterol, good source of fiber	Contains gluten
Starch:				
Potatoes ✓	Avoid pesticides by going organic.	OK	Antioxidant rich, Lowers Blood Pressure	
Snacks & Bakery:				
50% cracked wheat kernel bread		NO		Contains gluten
Bagel, white, frozen		NO		Contains trans fats and can increase cholesterol, may contain excess sugar and salt.

Food	Tips	Eat	The Good	The Bad
Baguette, white, plain		NO		Contains gluten
Coarse barley bread, 75-80% kernels		OK		
Corn chips, plain, salted	✓	Mode rately		
Corn tortilla	✓	Eat mode rately		
Fast Food Pizza (baked dough, cheese and tomato)		NO		Contains gluten
Fruit Roll-Ups®		NO		
Graham crackers		NO		Contain gluten
Hamburger bun	Choose whole grains. ✓	Eat mode rately		Contains gluten
Kaiser roll		NO		Contains gluten
M & M's®, peanut		Eat mode rately		
Air Popped popcorn, plain ✓	Choose unbuttered, low salt varieties.	OK		Artificial butter flavor contains toxic chemicals.
Pita bread, white ✓	Best if whole wheat.	OK		Contains gluten

Food	Tips	Eat	The Good	The Bad
Potato chips		NO		Contains trans fats and can increase bad cholesterol, may contain excess sugar and salt.
Pretzels, oven-baked		NO		Contains trans fats and can increase bad cholesterol, may contain excess sugar and salt.
Pumpernick el bread	✓	Eat Mode rately		
Rice cakes		NO		Contains trans fats and can increase bad cholesterol, may contain excess sugar and salt.
Rye crisps		NO		
Shortbread		NO		
Snickers Bar®		NO		
Soda crackers		NO		
Sponge cake, plain		Eat mode rately		Have trans fats that increase LDL Cholesterol. May contain too much sugar or salt.

Food	Tips	Eat	The Good	The Bad
Vanilla cake made from packet mix with vanilla frosting (Betty Crocker)		NO		Contains trans fats and can increase bad cholesterol, may contain excess sugar and salt.
Vanilla wafers		NO		Contains trans fats and can increase bad cholesterol, may contain excess sugar and salt.
Waffles, Aunt Jemima (Quaker Oats)	Choose whole grain varieties	NO		Contains trans fats and can increase bad cholesterol, may contain excess sugar and salt.
Wheat tortilla	Choose whole grain varieties	Eat moderately		Contains gluten
White wheat flour bread	Eat less than once a week	NO		High glycemic index, low fiber, check label as some brands contain too much salt
Whole wheat bread ✓		OK	High in antioxidants and fiber, revs up metabolism and lowers cholesterol.	Contains gluten
Wonder™ bread		NO		

Food	Tips	Eat	The Good	The Bad
Sweets & Sweeteners:				
Brown Sugar	✓	Eat moderately	Higher nutrient content than white sugar.	
Candies		NO		No nutritional value
Chocolate	✓	Eat moderately		Contains sugar and fat, may aggravate acid reflux.
Dark Chocolate (+ 60%)	Avoid eating with milk. ✓	OK	Antioxidant, good for heart health	May aggravate acid reflux.
Honey	✓	Eat moderately	High in nutrients, low in sugar	Calorie content similar to sugar
Jelly Beans		NO		
Marmalade (+ 65% fruit)	✓	Eat moderately		Check label for sugar content
Nutella		NO		Watch sugar and fat content
Raw Cane Sugar		Eat moderately	Is a better option than white sugar. Has more minerals and vitamins.	
Artificial Sweeteners: Stevia, Splenda, Nutrsweet.	Controversy over Splenda's possible toxicity.	NO		

Food	Tips	Eat	The Good	The Bad
White Sugar		NO		No nutritional value
Drinks & Beverages:				
Alcoholics (Beer, Liquors, Red Wine, Champagne) ✓	Limit to two servings per day for men, one a day for women.	Drink moderately red wine.	Red Wine is Anti-inflammatory and rich in resveratrol and other antioxidants, protects the brain.	May aggravate acid reflux.
Coconut Milk		NO		High in saturated fat, may raise LDL Cholesterol
Diet Soda		NO		May aggravate acid reflux. Many contain artificial sweeteners, which may be toxic.
100% Fruit Juices (Lemon, Cranberry, Pineapple, Grape, Carrots, Blueberries, Apple, Pomegranate)	Watch for added sugars ✓	OK	High in antioxidants, Protects brain and heart	May contain added sugar. Tomato juice may aggravate acid reflux.
Italian Coffee		OK	Antioxidant	May aggravate acid reflux.

Food	Tips	Eat	The Good	The Bad
Soft Drinks (Coke, Fanta, Gatorade)		NO		Too much sugar and may aggravate acid reflux.
Teas or Herbal Infusions ✓	e.g. mint or chamomile and green tea are good.	OK	High in Antioxidants, Lowers Cholesterol and Blood Pressure.	
Water ✓		OK		Bottled water may contain BPA. Tap Water may contain nitrates and pesticides residues. Opt for filtered tap water.

Food	Tips	Eat	The Good	The Bad
Beans and Legumes:				
Beans (All) ✓	Great alternative to meat. Soak overnight to remove compounds that can cause gas. Simmer on the stove for an hour to an hour and a half, or cook in pressure cooker at 15 lb for 5-8 minutes. Add grains for complete protein. Cook a large batch and freeze the leftovers.	OK	Revs up metabolism, lowers blood pressure and cholesterol, great source of fiber, calcium, iron, and B vitamins.	Canned beans may contain added salt and sugar.
Garbanzo Beans (Chickpeas) ✓	Same as above.	OK	Revs up metabolism, lowers blood pressure and cholesterol, great source of fiber, calcium, iron, and B vitamins.	Canned beans may contain added salt and sugar.
Lentils ✓	Simmer on the stove for an hour to 30-40 minutes. Add grains for complete protein. Cook a large batch and freeze the leftovers.	OK	Revs up metabolism, lowers blood pressure and cholesterol, great source of fiber, calcium, iron, and B vitamins.	Canned beans may contain added salt and sugar.

Food	Tips	Eat	The Good	The Bad
Peanut Butter ✓	Choose natural peanut butter to avoid trans fats while satisfying sugar cravings. Try on celery sticks for added fiber.	OK	Monounsaturated fats lower bad cholesterol, also high in B vitamins.	Watch for trans fats
Peanuts ✓	Great for snacking	OK	Revs up metabolism, Monounsaturated fats lower bad cholesterol, also high in B vitamins, iron, and calcium	
Peas ✓	No need to soak, simmer an hour to an hour and a half.	OK	Antioxidant	Canned beans may contain added salt and sugar.
Soy foods (e.g. tofu) ?		OK	Revs up metabolism, Omega-3 fatty acids lower bad cholesterol, lowers blood pressure, also high in B vitamins, iron, and calcium	

Food	Tips	Eat	The Good	The Bad
Soybeans	Great alternative to meat. Soak overnight to remove compounds that can cause gas. Simmer on the stove for an hour to an hour and a half, or cook in pressure cooker at 15 lb for 5-8 minutes. Add grains for complete protein. Cook a large batch and freeze the leftovers.	OK	Revs up metabolism, Omega-3 fatty acids lower bad cholesterol, lowers blood pressure, also high in B vitamins, iron, and calcium	
Vegetables:				
Artichokes		OK	Anti-inflammatory, Antioxidant, Prebiotics nourish beneficial gut bacteria	
Asparagus	✓	OK		
Beets	✓	OK	Revs up metabolism, Rich in antioxidants and folate	
Bell Peppers	✓ Avoid pesticides by going organic.	OK	Antioxidant	
Broccoli	Buy local and in season. Wash before eating and eat within 2-3 days. Good on salad.	OK	High in calcium, iron, folic acid, and antioxidants, anti-Inflammatory, lowers blood pressure	

Food	Tips	Eat	The Good	The Bad
Brussels Sprouts ✓	Buy local and in season. Wash before eating and eat within 2-3 days. Good on salad..	OK	High in calcium, iron, folic acid, and antioxidants, anti-Inflammatory, lowers blood pressure	
Cabbage ✓		OK	Antioxidant	
Capers ✓		OK	Antioxidant	
Carrots ✓	Buy local and in season. Wash before eating and eat within 2-3 days. Good on salad.	OK	High in antioxidants, lowers blood pressure	
Cauliflowers ✓	Buy local and in season. Wash before eating and eat within 2-3 days. Good on salad.	OK	High in calcium, iron, folic acid, and antioxidants, anti-Inflammatory, lowers blood pressure	
Celery ✓		OK	Anti-inflammatory and antioxidant	
Eggplants		OK	Antioxidant	
Fennel		OK	Low calorie and High in fiber	
Green Pepper ✓		OK	Anti-inflammatory and antioxidant	
Kale ?		OK	Revs up metabolism, high in calcium, folate, and antioxidants.	
Lettuce ✓	Avoid pesticides by going organic.	OK	Antioxidant	

Food	Tips	Eat	The Good	The Bad
Olives ✓		OK	Have Monounsaturated fats that decrease LDL without decreasing HDL	Watch for added salt.
Onions ✓		OK	Lower Blood Pressure, Protect the Heart	May aggravate acid reflux.
Pumpkins	Buy local and in season. Wash before eating and eat within 2-3 days. Good on salad.	OK	Antioxidant	
Radicchio ✓		OK		
Red Pepper ✓		OK	Anti-inflammatory and antioxidant	
Spinaches ✓	Buy local and in season. Wash before eating and eat within 2-3 days. Good on salad. Avoid pesticides by going organic.	OK	Anti-inflammatory and antioxidant, revs up metabolism, good source of folate, protects against macular degeneration.	
Squash ✓		OK	Antioxidant	
Sweet Potatoes ✓		OK	Antioxidant	
Tomatoes ✓	Buy local and in season. Wash before eating and eat within 2-3 days. Good on salad.	OK	High in lycopene and other antioxidants, Heart Healthy	Watch for added sodium. May aggravate acid reflux.

Food	Tips	Eat	The Good	The Bad
Turnip Tops		OK	Revs up metabolism, high in antioxidants and folate.	
Zucchini ✓		OK	Antioxidant	
Milk and Dairy:				
Almond Milk	Good milk substitute. Add dark chocolate powder or coffee for flavor. Good in smoothies	OK	Lower LDL Cholesterol, Rich in fiber and Calcium	Watch for added sugar, oil and salt.
Butter	Limit consumption, olive oil is a good substitute	NO		Contains saturated and trans fats that can raise bad cholesterol.
Cheese (Creamy, Ricotta, Mozzarella, Parmesan, Feta)	Ricotta has the lowest fat amount.	Eat Moderately	High in calcium and Vitamins A, B12, and D	Contains saturated and trans fats that can raise bad cholesterol.
Cream (Coffee)	Consume sparingly	NO		Contains saturated and trans fats that can raise bad cholesterol.

Food	Tips	Eat	The Good	The Bad
Milk (Cow, Sheep, Goat)	Consume sparingly	Drink Moderately	High in calcium and Vitamins B12 and D	Contains fats that can raise cholesterol. May increase production of IGF-1 hormone. Does not protect against osteoporosis
Oat Milk	Good milk substitute. Add dark chocolate powder or coffee for flavor. Good in smoothies	OK	High in fiber and folic acid and low in bad cholesterol	Watch for added sugar, oil and salt.
Processed Cheese		NO		Watch for added salt.
Rice Milk	Good milk substitute. Add dark chocolate powder or coffee for flavor. Good in smoothies	OK	Low fat contents	Watch for added sugar, oil and salt.
Soy Milk	Very good milk and eggs substitute in recipes. Watch if it's GMO	OK		Watch for added sugar, oil and salt.
Margarine	Easier to spread, no trans fats.	NO		Contains saturated and trans fats that raise LDL Cholesterol
Yogurt		Eat moderately	Probiotic	Watch for added sugar.

Food	Tips	Eat	The Good	The Bad
Meat & Fish:				
Cod	Contains less mercury than other fish. Okay to eat 2-3 times a week.	OK	Low fat, lower risk of mercury contamination	
Mackerel	Look for varieties packed in water, avoid smoked. Contains low mercury.	OK	High in Iron, Selenium, Vitamins B12, B6 and D; Contains Omega-3 fatty acids that improves both HDL and LDL.	If canned, watch for added sodium
Poultry ✓	Eat 2-3 times a week.	OK	High in Iron and Vitamins B12 and B6. Lean and Healthier than many other kinds of meat.	
Processed Meats (Ham, Sausages, Salami, Bologna)	Avoid or limit to occasional consumption	NO		Contains saturated fats that increase LDL Cholesterol. Contains nitrates and too much sodium.
Red Meats (Veal, Beef, Pork, Buffalo, Goat, Sheep, Lamb) and Game	Eat 2-3 times a month.	Eat lean cuts in moderation.	High in Iron, Selenium, and Vitamins B12 and B6	Contains saturated fats that increase LDL Cholesterol. Contains nitrates and too much sodium. Cook well done, but avoid excessively high temperatures

Food	Tips	Eat	The Good	The Bad
Salmon	Consume once a week or less and avoid smoked. ✓	OK	High in Iron, Selenium, Vitamins B12, B6 and D; Contains Omega-3 fatty acids that improves both HDL and LDL.	If canned, watch for added sodium. May contain mercury.
Sardines ✓	Contain a reduced amount of mercury than other fish. May eat 2-3 times a week.	OK	High in Iron, Selenium, Vitamins B12, B6 and D; Contains Omega-3 fatty acids that improves both HDL and LDL.	If canned, watch for added sodium.
Shellfish (Clams, Oysters)	Consume once a week or less.	OK	High in Iron, Selenium, Vitamins B12, B6 and D; Contains Omega-3 fatty acids that improves both HDL and LDL.	
Shrimp ✓	May eat 2-3 times a week.	OK	High in Vitamin B12 and Calcium. Less mercury than some other kinds of seafood	High in Cholesterol
Swordfish	Consume once a week or less and avoid smoked.	OK		Contains mercury

Food	Tips	Eat OK	The Good	The Bad
Tuna ✓	Look for packed in water and avoid smoked. Eat less than once a week.	OK	High in Iron, Selenium, Vitamins B12, B6 and D; Contains Omega-3 fatty acids that improves both HDL and LDL.	If canned watch for added sodium. May contain mercury
Oils:				
Canola Oil ✓		OK	Antioxidant; Has Polyunsaturated, Monounsaturated fats and Omega-3 fatty acids that improve cholesterol levels	
Coconut Oil	Avoid	NO		Has saturated fats that raise LDL Cholesterol
Corn Oil	Do not use for frying.	NO	Antioxidant; Has Polyunsaturated fats that decrease LDL	Lowers HDL
Extra Virgin Olive Oil ✓	Best for seasoning. Limit to 2 tbps. a day. Look for "Cold pressed". Good substitute for butter.	OK	Contains antioxidants and Monounsaturated fats improve cholesterol levels	
Flaxseed Oil		OK	Contains antioxidants and Omega-3 fatty acids that improve cholesterol levels	
Palm Oil	Avoid	NO		Contains saturated fats that raises LDL Cholesterol

Food	Tips	Eat	The Good	The Bad
Sunflower Oil	Not good for frying or seasoning hot dishes.	NO	Contains antioxidants and polyunsaturated fats improve cholesterol levels	Lowers HDL
Nuts and Seeds:				
Almonds	Good for snacking. Avoid salted. ✓	OK	Revs up metabolism, high in calcium and antioxidants, contains polyunsaturated and monounsaturated fats that improve cholesterol levels	Watch calorie content and possible added salt.
Chestnuts		OK	High in protein, iron, calcium, and antioxidants, has anti-inflammatory properties, lowers cholesterol	Watch calorie content
Flaxseed		OK	High in antioxidants and Omega-3	Watch calorie content
Pine Nuts		OK	High in protein, iron, calcium, and antioxidants, Anti Inflammatory, lowers cholesterol	Watch calorie content
Pistachio ✓	Good for snacking, look for unsalted.	OK	High in protein, iron, calcium, and antioxidants, Anti Inflammatory, lowers cholesterol	Watch calorie content and possible added salt.
Pumpkin Seeds ✓	Good for snacking, look for unsalted.	OK	High in protein, iron, calcium, and antioxidants, Anti Inflammatory, lowers cholesterol	Watch calorie content and possible added salt.

Food	Tips	Eat	The Good	The Bad
Sesame seeds		OK	High in protein and fiber	
Sunflower Seeds ✓	Good for snacking, look for unsalted.	OK	High in antioxidants; Contains polyunsaturated fats that lower LDL	
Walnuts ✓	Good for snacking, look for unsalted.	OK	Revs up metabolism, High in antioxidants; Contains polyunsaturated fats and Omega-3 fatty acids that improve cholesterol levels	
Eggs ✓	Immerse in cold salted water and if it sinks it's fresh! Do not wash.	Eat moderately	High in iron and Vitamins B12, A and D	Yolks are high in cholesterol. Limit to 2 a week.
Mushrooms ✓		OK	Low calories	
Herbs - Spices - Condiments:				
Allaurum	Makes beans easier to digest	OK	Helps Digestion	
Basil	Good in Pesto sauce.	OK	Anti-inflammatory and high in antioxidants	
Chili ✓		OK	High in Antioxidants, dilates the blood vessels	Can aggravate acid reflux.
Cider Vinegar ✓		OK	Anti-inflammatory and high in antioxidants	Acidic, may alter gut bacteria
Cinnamon ✓		OK		

Food	Tips	Eat	The Good	The Bad
Garlic ✓		OK	Lowers blood pressure and protects the heart	
Ginger ✓		OK	High in Vitamin C and other antioxidants	
Ketchup	Limit to once a week ✓	Eat moderately	High in lycopene	Watch for added sugar and sodium
Liquorices		OK	Aids digestion, diuretic	
Marjoram	Good for flavoring fish and meats.	OK		
Mayonnaise	Look for fat free. ✓	Eat Moderately		High in fat
Mint		OK	Anti-inflammatory and high in antioxidants, aids digestion	Can aggravate acid reflux.
Mustard ✓		Eat moderately		Acidic
Oregano	Good on Pizza.	OK		
Parsley	Good with fish.	OK	High in vitamin C and calcium	
Rosemary	Good with meats and fish.	OK	Aids digestion	
Saffron		OK		
Sage		OK		

Food	Tips	Eat	The Good	The Bad
Salt	Raw unrefined sea salt contains a variety of minerals, making it a healthier option. Cut salt by half and combine with some herbs or sesame seeds to limit consumption without sacrificing flavor	NO		High in sodium, may .raise blood press and can stomach cancer
Soy Sauce	✓	Eat moderately		High in sodium
Thyme	Good to flavor soups and sauces.	OK		
Vanilla		OK	Antioxidant	
Wine Vinegar and Balsamic	✓	OK	Aids Digestion	
Frozen Foods:				
Chicken Nuggets		OK		
Fish and Vegetables		OK	Freezing preserves some nutrients	Freezing destroys most of the omega-3 contents
Ice Cream	✓	Eat moderately		Watch the sugar and fat content.

Free radicals are atoms or groups of atoms with unpaired electrons. They are formed as a result of exposure to pollution or radiation as well as being a normal by-product of cellular activity. These unpaired electrons are highly reactive and cause damage to the cells that is associated with aging, cancer, and heart disease. Antioxidants are known to help stop free radicals and reduce the damage they cause.

There are hundreds of dietary sources of substances with antioxidant properties. Vitamins C and E, some forms of Vitamin A, and selenium have all been fairly thoroughly studied, though they are far from the only ones.

Sources of some antioxidants include:

- Vitamin C - Citrus fruits of all varieties, berries, broccoli, peppers, and tomatoes.
- Vitamin E – Almonds and other nuts, seeds, vegetable oils, leafy greens, gluten-free whole grains, fatty fish.
- Selenium - Meat, fish, whole-grain cereal, dairy products, Brazil nuts.
- Beta-carotene - Dark green, yellow, and orange fruits and vegetables (think carrots, oranges, squash, sweet potatoes, melon, tomatoes, and leafy greens).

Antioxidant Rich Substitutes

- Punch or soda – 100% fruit juice
- Bagels or donuts – whole-grain cereal with non-dairy milk
- Sugary cereal – oatmeal with non-dairy milk and topped with fruit
- Hamburger – turkey or veggie burger with lettuce and

tomato
- Peanut butter and jelly – natural peanut butter and fruit
- Deli Sandwich – grilled chicken sandwich or soup salad and whole grain bread
- Chips and dip – tortillas and salsa
- Chips – fruit, nuts, or raw vegetables
- Spaghetti and meatballs – whole-grain spaghetti with marinara and veggies
- Iceberg lettuce – raw spinach or other dark, leafy greens
- Butter or margarine – nut butters
- Red meat – poultry or fish
- Ice cream – sorbet or fruit and yogurt smoothie

Ways to increase the nutrients in your diet

- Choose a dark green salad with lots of fresh veggies for lunch. Top with vinegar and oil or other low fat dressing.
- Top yogurt, cereal, or fruit with nuts for crunch, flavor and nutrients. They can be high in fat, so go easy.
- Serve two or more vegetables with dinner. Stir fry is a flavorful way to get plenty of vegetables at once.

You know calcium for strengthening bones and teeth, but it's also important in the transmission of signals in the nervous system, helping muscles to contract, and maintaining proper blood pH.

When blood does not contain enough calcium for these processes, calcium is pulled from the bones. Lack of calcium contributes to weak bones and osteoporosis.

If you ask many people what foods are good sources of calcium, most of them will tell you dairy foods. In fact, many plant foods are great sources of calcium. Some may not contain quite as much as dairy, while some (such as spinach) contain much more. A diet rich in a variety of calcium rich fruits and vegetables provides plenty of calcium.

Calcium rich fruits and vegetables have the added benefit of also being rich in fiber and a variety antioxidants and other nutrients.

Ways to increase your calcium intake include:

- Soy foods – Fortified soymilk contains a lot of calcium
- Vegetables – ½ cup collard greens, kale, or broccoli
- Fruit – 5 dried figs, 1 orange, or a cup of fortified orange juice
- Nuts and seeds – 1 oz sesame seeds or 2 tablespoons of almonds
- Grains – 1 tortilla
- Fish – 2 sardines or 3 oz canned salmon with bones

Eggshell is an excellent source of calcium. Soak an egg in lemon juice overnight, remove, and add a teaspoonful to a glass of warm water. The acid in the lemon juice dissolves the calcium.

If you're wondering what the big deal is about fiber, it turns out that it's a vital part of a healthy lifestyle. Consuming adequate fiber has a variety of health benefits, including stimulating digestion, lowering cholesterol, and aiding in weight loss.

The modern diet that most people consume only provides about half the fiber needed for good health. Men should try to consume at least 38 grams per day, while women should aim for 25 grams per day.

The best sources of fiber are gluten-free whole grains, especially barley and brown rice. Other good sources are dried fruits, especially dried figs and raisins, peas, almonds, and legumes. Most fruits and vegetables are also great sources of fiber.

What is it?

Fiber is indigestible component of plant foods. There are a variety of different types of fiber, categorized into soluble and insoluble.

Soluble fiber absorbs moisture in the digestive tract and takes on a gel-like consistency. This gel slows digestion and regulates levels of glucose and insulin. Soluble fiber also ferments in the colon, creating substances the promote colon health.

Insoluble fiber does not absorb water, but does add bulk, which has a laxative effect.

Health benefits of fiber

- Digestion – Insoluble fiber prevents or eases constipation, hemorrhoids, diverticulosis, and other diseases of the digestive tract.

- Heart – Soluble fiber lowers cholesterol and insulin levels. Diets high in fiber may help lower bad cholesterol and raise good cholesterol
- Diabetes – High fiber diets decrease the risk of type 2 diabetes. For those with diabetes, soluble fiber can help regulate sugar levels, reducing the risk of complications from the disease.
- Cancer – A number of studies have shown that consistently consuming adequate fiber may reduce risk of certain cancers, particularly colon, prostate, and breast. It's possible that it's not so much the fiber that reduces the risk, but other components of foods that are typically higher in fiber, or even an interaction between fiber and other nutrients in the foods. Either way, this is a great reason to focus on whole foods rather than trying to supplement your diet with pills.
- Weight management – High fiber foods provide bulk in the digestive tract, helping you to feel full longer. It also moderates sugar levels, helping to reduce cravings.

Here are some easy ways to get more fiber:

- Include gluten-free whole grain cereal as part of your breakfast. Mix in some fresh or dried fruit. Substitute an orange for orange juice.
- Opt for higher fiber snacks such as popcorn or fruit.
- Much of the fiber in fruits and vegetables is found in the peel, so leave it on. Be sure to scrub them thoroughly to remove any pesticides or other chemicals.
- Add more vegetables and legumes to soups, stews salads and casseroles.
- As much as possible, eat more whole foods than processed foods.
- Swap fresh fruit for sugary desserts after dinner. You

might be surprised at how easily your family makes the switch.

How to Get Enough Folate

Folate, also known as folic acid, folacin, or Vitamin B9, is vital to the synthesis of DNA and RNA. Folate deficiency is associated with several health complications, including megaloblastic anemia, a form of anemia that causes red blood cells to grow too large because they are unable to divide.

Other health benefits of folate include:

- Reduced risk of birth defects – Women who are pregnant or could become pregnant should ensure they consume enough folate to protect against neural tube defects such as spina bifida. All prenatal vitamins contain the nutrient and all women of child-bearing age are encouraged to make sure they are getting enough of the nutrient, as these birth defects occur very early in pregnancy, often before a woman finds out she is pregnant.
- Heart health – Getting enough folate reduces the amount of homocysteine in the blood. Excess homocysteine has been linked to an increased risk of cardiovascular disease.
- Colon health – A Nurse's Healthy study found that women who had consumed at least 400mcg of folate each day over time had a significantly lower incidence of colon cancer.
- Brain health – Research has found a correlation between inadequate folate levels in the elderly and increased risk of depression, dementia, and cognitive difficulties.

Ways to make sure you're getting enough folate:

- Eat a healthy breakfast with fortified cereal. Add a handful of berries or half banana sliced.
- Drink a glass of fortified orange juice with breakfast.
- Enjoy a salad filled with dark leafy green vegetables.
- Toss some legumes into soup, salad, or casserole.
- Snack on peanut butter and gluten-free, whole-grain crackers or bread.
- Mix together salsa with diced fresh peaches to top fish, poultry, or grilled vegetables.
- Cut some bananas in half, freeze them, and dip in melted dark chocolate. For an added nutritional punch, roll in some chopped pecans for a gourmet dessert.
- Watch for store specials on berries and stock up. Enjoy a handful and freeze the extra to blend with non-dairy milk for nutritious smoothie. This can also help you satisfy your sweet tooth.
- Cut watermelon into shapes and freeze on a tray. Once frozen, put them in an airtight container and store in the freezer to eat like a Popsicle.
- Add fresh fruit to cereal and yogurt for breakfast on the go.

For many people, the biggest obstacle to healthy eating is time. However, eating healthy does not require spending hours in the kitchen. The key to healthier meals in less time is smart shopping and having the right ingredients available.

Here are some tips and tricks to help you improve the nutrition in your meals:

- in the freezer - the freezer section at your local grocery store is packed with a variety of fruits and vegetables. Stir fry blends and other mixed vegetables make preparing a nutritious meal quick and simple. Stock up on these to use when your supply of fresh produce is running low. Beware that frozen meals often have added sodium and fat, so be sure to read the label and look for products without added ingredients. Some of the best choices include:
    - Festive medley – This mix typically contains kidney beans which are high in protein.
    - Chopped onions – A great way to save time and tears.
    - Frozen peppers – Very colorful and a great addition to soups, chilies, or pasta.
    - French fries – precut fries are easy to bake and can be served with sandwiches, chicken, fish, or veggie burgers. Look for low-fat products that are unseasoned. Seasoned frozen fries typically contain added sodium.
- In the produce aisle – Preparing your own produce saves money, but prepackaged produce can save you a great deal of time. Some good choices include:
    - Stir Fry medley – All the veggies you need for a great stir fry, precut and ready to go.

- Salad mixes – A basic salad in a bag, prewashed and ready dish up, dress, and eat.
- Salad bar – Some stores have a salad bar with all the fixings washed, cut and ready to assemble just the way you like it.
- Baby carrots – Baby carrots aren't actually immature carrots, they're imperfect carrots that have been cut down to make them more attractive. They're great as a garnish or for eating right out of the bag. Be sure to look for organic baby carrots, as some brands are washed in chlorine.
- Minced garlic – Garlic is a superfood, containing compounds that are great for boosting the immune system and overall health. Add just a bit of minced garlic to add flavor to nearly any food.
- Seasoning – Seasoning mixes save not only time, but money as well. Instead of buying and measuring several different spices, simply scoop a perfectly proportioned mix. Watch the labels for added salt. Here are some great ones:
  - Italian seasoning – Consisting primarily of basil, oregano, and marjoram, Italian seasoning is especially good in soup, pasta, and chili.
  - Lemon pepper –A great addition to poultry, fish, baked potato, salad, or vegetables.
  - Cajun seasoning –Cajun is good on poultry, fish, and French fries.
  - Garlic parsley – Adds a zesty green flavor to pasta, poultry, fish, and salad.
  - Chili powder – Consisting of ground chili peppers, cumin, and garlic. Use it to add head to rice, poultry, and soup.
  - Apple pie spice – Quench your sweet tooth by adding this mix to baked apples, fruit salad, applesauce, yogurt, or coffee.

- Pumpkin pie spice – Add flavor to winter squash, fruits, and baked goods.
- All-purpose herbs – Not exactly a mix, but parsley, thyme and a bay leaf are a good combination for many foods. Known as a bouquet garni in French, the combination is a staple in French cuisine. Add a few cloves for sweet heat, or a bit of citrus zest for meaty stews and braises. Throw in a bit of rosemary, sage, or savory for a Mediterranean flavor. A garlic clove is a good addition for many foods. If you have a green thumb, try growing some of these yourself, and tie bunches of them together to store in a cool, dry place for easy use.

Herbs and Spices Recipes

To make your own spice mixes, try some of the following recipes:

Stir Fry Mix

This mix adds flavor to any stir-fry.

- 1 Tbsp. ground ginger
- Generous pinch of ground cloves
- 2 Tbsp. garlic powder
- 1 tsp. red pepper flakes

Combine ingredients and store at room temperature in an airtight container.

Italian Seasoning

Add authentic Italian flavor to pasta, salad, or soup, it's a delicious addition for garlic toast. Add approximately 1 teaspoon for every 4 servings of pasta about ten minutes before it's finished.

- 3 Tbsp. dried oregano
- 3 Tbsp. dried basil
- 2 Tbsp. dried marjoram
- 1 Tbsp. garlic powder
- 1 tsp. dried thyme

Combine ingredients and store at room temperature in an airtight container.

Sweet Spice

Adds a sweet spiciness to fruit salads, cereal, and yogurt.

- 2 Tbsp. ground cinnamon
- 1 Tbsp. ground ginger
- 1/2 Tbsp. ground nutmeg
- 1 tsp. allspice
- Pinch ground cloves

Combine ingredients and store at room temperature in an airtight container. You may want to use a shaker container with this mix.

Rice Pilaf Seasoning

Add flavor to rice pilaf, stuffing, and cornbread, or add to bread mixes for a distinct flavor. Use about 1 teaspoon of mix for every four servings.

- 1 Tbsp. oregano
- 1 tsp. dried ground sage
- 1 tsp. dried rosemary, crushed
- 2 tsp. onion powder
- 1 tsp. garlic powder

Combine ingredients and store at room temperature in an airtight container.

Chili Mix

Add heat to dips, salads, baked potatoes, chili, and pasta.

- 3 Tbsp. ground pure red chili powder
- 1 Tbsp. garlic powder
- 1 Tbsp. cumin
- 1 Tbsp. dried oregano

Combine ingredients and store at room temperature in an airtight container. Try toasting the chili powder and cumin in a warm skillet or saute pan to bring out their flavor. How much to use depends on how spicy you like your food. Start with a teaspoon for every six servings, and adjust to taste.

Preparing healthy meals starts with being smart in the grocery store. How you shop directly influences both your eating habits and how nutritious your meals are. Every decision you make at the grocery store either supports or undermines your goals. This is why it's vital that you know how to evaluate the nutritional value of the food you buy.

What to look for on the label:

- Fat calories – It is recommended that you limit your calories from fat to 30% of your total calories for the day. Focus on foods that have less than 30% of calories from fat and this goal will be easier to achieve.
- Saturated fat – This type of fat is the type that is responsible for clogged arteries. You should limit your saturated fat to no more than 10% of your daily calories. Look for foods with less than 2g of saturated fat per serving.
- Sodium – Excess sodium can raise your blood pressure and experts recommend limiting your intake to no more than 1500mg per day. Look for foods that contain 5% or less of the recommended daily limits per serving.

Tips for getting the best produce

Fresh produce can be expensive, and you want to get the best you can for your money. How do you find the best pieces? Look for the following:

- Vivid color – In most cases, you want to look for fruits and vegetables that are brightly colored. Look for signs of wilting, discoloration, or brown spots. When buying leafy green vegetables, look for crisp leaves.

- Firm– Avoid produce with mushy spots. If you get home and you find a bad spot, cut around it.
- Heavy for size – The heavier the vegetable or piece of fruit is, the juicier and more flavorful it will be. Lightweight fruits may be dry and lacking in flavor.
- Aroma – Smell the produce, especially melons. They should have a fruity aroma. Don't be embarrassed to sniff your fruits and veggies, it's a great way to test freshness.

Boost Your Immunity with Fruits and Vegetables

Fruits and vegetables are packed with vitamins, minerals, and fiber, along with hundreds of phytochemicals with antioxidant, anti-inflammatory, and immune boosting properties. Here are some things you may not have known:

- Asparagus is a good source of folate, which can lower your risk of heart disease. If you are considering adding to your family, it can also reduce the risk of birth defects.
- Avocadoes are rich in heart-healthy fats. Keep in mind that even heart-healthy fat can compromise your weight loss goals, so go easy.
- Berries contain ellagic acid, a phytochemical that can lower cancer risk.
- Garlic and onions contain allicin, an immune boosting phytochemical that can reduce the risk of cancer and heart disease.
- Oranges contain limonene, a phytochemical that may be able to lower the risk of cancer and heart disease.
- Sweet potatoes are rich in antioxidants that can lower the risk of certain cancer and slow aging.
- Tomatoes are a great source of lycopene, a heart-healthy phytochemical that can reduce the risk of certain cancers.

Cooking tomato-based foods in cast iron cookware can increase the iron content of the food.

Choose the Best Protein

Many high-protein foods, especially animal proteins, also happen to be high in fat. Look for lean cuts and remove skin from poultry to help you achieve your healthy lifestyle goals. Choose fish, turkey or chicken breast, or other white meat poultry. Here are some tips to get the most protein with the least fat:

- Trim visible fat. When choosing a cut of meat some marbling will impart flavor and tenderness to the meat, but keep in mind that marbling is fat, so go easy.
- When buying canned tuna, salmon, chicken, or other meat, look for products that are packed in water instead of oil, and check the label for added salt.
- Fatty, cold-water fish such as trout, salmon, albacore tuna, sardines, and mackerel are all good sources of omega-3 fatty acids, which lower LDL cholesterol and promote heart and brain health.

Healthy Grains

Packed with fiber, whole grains can help improve digestion, lower cholesterol, regulate blood sugar levels, and reduce the risk of certain cancers. Which ones are the best?

The best choices are brown rice, oatmeal, barley, quinoa, bulgur, and grits. These are all low in fat, and typically do not contain added sugar. However, beware of instant cereals and packaged mixes that can have added sugar, fat, or salt.

Breads and packages cereals are often high in sugar and sodium.

Check the label and look for gluten-free whole-grain varieties. Look for products with at least 5g of fiber per serving and whole-grain as a main ingredient. Be sure to check the sodium content as well.

The following whole grains are inexpensive, easy to prepare, and high in fiber:

- 2/3 cup cooked oatmeal – 6g
- 1/2 cup cooked brown rice – 2.5g
- 1 cup cooked quinoa – 2g
- 1 cup air-popped popcorn – 2g

Groceries are not cheap, and prices keep rising. Healthy food may be more expensive than packaged processed foods, but you don't have to sacrifice nutrition to save money.

Beans, whole grains, and in season fruits and vegetables are some of the least expensive and healthiest food you can buy. These foods are high in fiber and low in saturated fat and sodium than processed foods, baked goods, crackers, chips, or desserts.

Save Time and Money by Planning Ahead

Every week, most people eat 7 breakfasts, lunches and dinners. Many people add a snack or two each day. This comes to 21 meals and several snacks every week, or 1,095 meals, plus snacks, each year. Multiply this by the number of people in your household, and you're talking about a lot of food.

By planning your meals and snacks a week ahead, you can both time and money. It is less expensive to prepare dinner than to go to a restaurant. By planning before you go shopping, you'll be sure to get everything you need (no last minute runs after something you forgot), and not fill your cart with impulse buys.

You can easily save thousands of dollars a year just by spending a few minutes to plan what you're going to eat each week. Don't feel like you're locked in once you have your meals planned. If something comes up and you don't have the time for what you had planned this evening, or if you are just in the mood for whatever you had planned for tomorrow, switch it around.

Here are some ways to save even more on groceries:

- Shop less frequently – Shopping once a week or even less

will save on not only groceries, but also on fuel. The less often you go, the less often you will encounter the temptation to buy stuff you don't need.

- Limit processed foods – When you buy unprocessed or minimally processed foods, you'll save money and improve the nutrition value of your food. For example, a bag of potatoes are significantly cheaper per ounce than a bag of French fries, and contains significantly less fat and sodium.
- Stock up on frozen foods and nonperishables when they are on sale – These items last much longer and are typically less expensive than refrigerated foods. By stocking up on these things when they are on sale, you not only save money, but future shopping trips are faster because you really only need to pick up fresh produce and refrigerated goods. Here are some items to consider stocking:
  - In the pantry:
    - Water-packed tuna
    - Lentils
    - Oatmeal
    - Pasta sauce
    - Natural peanut butter
    - Rice and brown rice
    - Soups
  - In the freezer:
    - Gluten-free whole-grain bread (gluten-free, whole grain)
    - Chicken
    - Egg whites
    - Unbreaded fish and seafood (check label, especially if seasoned)
    - Fruits

- Seafood
- Turkey
- Vegetables
- Base Meals around Produce – This is a great way to plan nutritious and inexpensive meals. Look at sales ads and plan around what is on sale. Produce that is in season is also generally less expensive than produce that must be shipped in from overseas. Come up with a few good dinners and make enough to have leftovers, and you should have a nice, healthy week.

At a loss for meal ideas? Consider some of the following:

- Zucchini, green beans, or other green vegetable with baked fish and rice
- Steam broccoli, zucchini, or green beans, or bake winter squash or spaghetti squash to have chicken or turkey breast.
- Make a salsa for burritos, tacos, chicken, fish, or as a dip for veggies and tortillas.
- Use up veggies left at the end of the week with a stir fry, casserole, or other dish. Consider carrots, mushrooms, spinach, and peppers.
- Salad
- Top cereal or yogurt with fruit for breakfast
- Have fruit for snacks and desserts
- Cole slaw made with oil and vinegar dressing and a pinch of oregano. A bit of crushed pineapple can add a tangy, sweet flavor.
- Risotto with veggies – Risotto is a creamy rice made with a short-grain rice known as Arborio rice. Add 3 cups of water to each cup of rice. Toss your veggies and seasonings in halfway through cooking. Stir well and serve hot.
- Turkey burger served on an English muffin or gluten-free

whole-grain bun. Top with lettuce and tomato.
- Carrot sticks, rounds, or slivers for snacking.
- Oven roasted potato wedges, season to taste with one of the seasoning mix recipes above.

Healthy Ways to Reduce your Grocery Budget

- Oatmeal – Swap expensive boxed cereal for steel cut oatmeal and save nearly $100 per year per person. This trick will also help you consume less sugar and sodium and more soluble fiber. A tub of oatmeal costs about the same as a box of cereal, but contains approximately three times as many servings.
- Water – Skip the bottled water and buy a stainless steel water bottle and fill it with filtered tap water. Soda can run as high as $5.00 for a 12 pack, and having soda on hand makes water less desirable. Limiting soda to special occasions can save you hundred and cut your sugar consumption by several pounds per year. A filter and reusable water bottle cost much less than you will save on sugary beverages.
- Rice and Potatoes – Both rice and potatoes are easy and inexpensive to buy in bulk, easy to store, easy to prepare, versatile, and delicious. Go to your favorite recipe website to find new ways to prepare both of these filling foods.
- Lean poultry – Buying a whole chicken is the least expensive, but be prepared to spend some time cutting it up and portioning it out. Once this is done, however, there are many different things you can do with it. Do a search for "what to do with a whole chicken" for ideas. If you prefer not to do this, chicken breasts, chicken tenders, and lean ground turkey are all reasonably priced and easy to use.
- Fish, frozen or canned in water – Fish is a nutritious way to add great flavor to rice and salads. When buying canned, look for small cans to help with portion control. For better

selection, look in the freezer section. Keep added salt and fat low by choosing plain varieties and seasoning the fish yourself.

- Tea – Save money and added sugar by skipped the bottles of already brewed tea and buy tea bags and brew your own. Tea is a great alternative to soda and other sugary drinks, with an added benefit of being packed with antioxidant phytochemicals. Brewing your own allows you to tailor your beverage to your preferred strength.

Use Your Freezer to Help you Eat Well on a Budget

If you're like most people, you don't have a lot of time to prepare an elaborate meal, so you've turned to prepackaged foods. Returning to a healthy way of eating when you don't have time to cook can be a daunting proposition. It doesn't have to be this way if you make your freezer your partner in creating a healthy lifestyle.

How can your freezer help you? You've probably heard about people who spend an entire day prepping and cooking tons of food to store for later. You could do this, and it does work well, but there's an easier way. When you cook, simply make a double batch, and freeze the extra in portion-size containers for snacking, or to heat up again to eat later in the week.

Here are some things to do to make it easier:

- Clean your freezer – I'm going to go out on a limb and guess that your freezer is packed with freezer-burned foods that you'll never eat. The first thing you need to do is clean out your freezer to make room for new, healthy foods. Stay on top of it by cleaning it out once a month.
- Buy some freezer containers and bags to have ready to store your food. Use a dry erase marker to write on the container

what it contains and the date.

- When you cook a meal, make a double batch and freeze the extra in small portions. You can freeze peanut butter sandwiches, rice, soups, and stir fry. Not all foods freeze well, foods that don't include gravies thickened with cornstarch, fruits and vegetables with high water content, cooked potatoes, and some dairy products. Experiment and find out what works.
- Prevent foodborne illness – Cool your food in a shallow dish in the refrigerator immediately after cooking before portioning and freezing.

Eating at a restaurant used to be an occasional treat, but many families today fall back on eating out several times per week. At the same time, restaurant portions are growing. It's no wonder, then, that the rate of obesity is increasing at a rate similar to that of restaurant sales.

In fact, many people spend nearly twice as much on restaurant meals as they did a few decades ago. As computers become ubiquitous, people also engage in significantly less physical activity.

Granted, restaurant meals are only one piece of the obesity puzzle, but because of the number of meals eaten in restaurants, and the growing size of restaurant portions, it's an important piece.

The bottom line of eating healthy in a restaurant is the same as eating healthy at home, it boils down to awareness. Be aware of what and how much you're eating when you're out. It's fine to indulge when eating out if eating out happens only on special occasions, but doing this on a regular basis will undermine all of your efforts.

Here are some things to be especially wary of:

- Meat based entrees, especially red meat. Here are calorie counts of steaks served in many steak houses:
  - 14 oz. New York 819 calories
  - 12 oz. sirloin 877 calories
  - 12 oz. prime rib 1,445 calories
- Beverages – A 26 oz soda will run you about 330 calories, while a 35 oz soda will run you 430 calories, and every refill

adds up. Some milkshakes can run close to 1,000 calories, plus lots of fat and sugar. Creamy coffee drinks can add 500 calories. Stick with water to save money, calories, and sugar. Ask for lemon for flavor.

- Bread – Some restaurants bring a breadbasket to your table when you're seated, and offer unlimited bread while you wait for your meal. When you're hungry, it can be easy to chow down. If you're hungry, ask for a salad to help tide you over until your meal arrives.

- Portion sizes – Huge portions served in restaurants can be your downfall. A value meal at a fast food place can run you over 1,500 calories, the majority of your calories for the day. Order from the lunch or a la carte menu, or divide your meal before you start eating and set half aside to eat later.

- Dessert – Dessert can be the worst part of any restaurant meal, adding as many as 1,000 calories to your meal. Look for a lower calorie dessert, such as fruit salad or sorbet, or share one dessert between multiple people.

- All-you-can-eat buffets are great for enjoying a wide variety of food without spending a lot of money. Unfortunately, studies show that the wider the variety of food that is available, the more calories you will consume. Not only this, but many of the foods on the buffet line are high in sugar, fat, salt, and calories. Opt for an all-you-can-eat salad bar instead and choose low-fat dressing and toppings.

- Hunger can lead to overeating. Eat a bit of fruit or another low-fat snack before you go out to take the edge off. This will keep you from letting your hunger influence your decision making.

- Restaurants serve lots of foods that are either breaded, fried, or otherwise loaded with fat and calories. To illustrate this point, a 2oz serving of French fries gives you 174 calories, while a 2oz baked potato has less than a third of that, at 52 calories. When eating out, look for places that have a lot of baked and grilled items on the menu, and steer clear of ingredients with a lot of fat.

Eating Smart when Eating Out

Besides choosing lighter options, try some of these other healthy strategies:

- Opt for soups made with broth over creamy soups and chowders.
- If you're feeling adventurous, try some of the vegetarian options.
- Opt for grilled or baked seafood.
- When ordering salad, ask to have the dressing on the side.

Restaurants generally want to make you happy. If you can't find what you want on the menu, consider requesting the following the following changes:

- Make omelets from egg whites
- Leave out the butter or oil
- Serve sauces and dressings on the side
- Leave out fatty items such as cheese or bacon

Fast Food Cheat Sheet

Nutrition and fast food can seem like mutually exclusive ideas, but it's not completely impossible to find healthy options in fast food. Choose places that have nutrition information available and look for items that contain less than 600mg of sodium per serving and are low in calories, fat, and saturated fat.

Many people eat fast food on a weekly basis or more, and the calories and fat can add up and sabotage your efforts quickly.

Here are some healthy options to look for at ethnic restaurants:

Mexican – Choose corn tortillas over hard shells and steer clear of cheese and deep fried items.

Chinese – Avoid deep fried items, wonton skins, and fried rice. Look for vegetable based items served over steamed rice and consider sharing with a friend.

Italian – Marinara sauce is lower in fat and calories than alfredo. Limit how much garlic bread and pasta you eat. Eat just one slice of pizza with a large salad.

Eating on the Run

Next to eating out, eating on the run is one of the biggest pitfalls for people trying to get healthy. Convenience foods are often high in fat, salt and calories. Keep a roll of paper towels and some hand sanitizer for easy cleaning. Get a cooler or an insulated lunch bag and keep some of the following items packaged and ready to go in the refrigerator:

- Fresh veggies cut into bite-sized pieces. Keep a small container filled with vinaigrette or other low-fat dressing to go with it.
- Fresh fruit cut into bite-sized pieces such as pineapple, mango, melon, or apples, as well as grapes and berries.
- Low fat plain yogurt
- Dried fruit
- Homemade trail mix
- 100% fruit compote
- 100% fruit juice

Pack your own 100 calorie snack packs with:

- Cereal – some cereals contain an easy 100 calories per cup, but check the label.
- Fortune cookies – at 15 calories each, you can put seven in a bag
- Graham crackers – 60 calories per square
- Air popped Popcorn – at 25 calories per cup, it takes 4 cups to get you to 100 calories (skip the butter and go easy on the salt)
- Grapes – Depending on the size of the grapes, it takes 15-25
- Blueberries – 1 cup
- Strawberries – 10-15, again depending on size
- Banana
- Low calorie granola – ½ cup
- Hard candy – 5-8, depending on the candy

Sandwiches are quick and easy, but can easily sabotage your efforts. Here's how to make a healthier sandwich:

- Start with gluten-free whole grain bread.
- Choose chicken or roasted turkey breast instead of higher fat meats like bologna or ham.
- Once or twice a week, consider having canned tuna or salmon.
- Use ½ as much meat and add lettuce, tomato, and other veggies such as red onion, carrots, cucumbers, and spinach.
- Dress with light mayonnaise. Mustard is a low calorie option, but it can be high in sodium.
- Freeze your bread to make peanut butter easier to spread

Make a delicious, nutritious tuna salad sandwich:

2 Tablespoons light mayo
3oz low-sodium tuna in water
¼ cup Romaine lettuce

1/3 tomato

This tuna salad recipe not only tastes better than the classic recipe, but it is far more nutritious. It provides:

- Three times the magnesium
- More than double the potassium
- More than double the Vitamin E
- Adds the B vitamins thiamin, niacin, and folate.

Tuna salad isn't the only sandwich that can be made healthier, peanut butter can as well. Spread 1 tablespoon of natural peanut butter onto frozen bread and add banana slices in place of jelly. Making peanut butter sandwiches this way gives you:

- Three times the Vitamin E
- Nearly double the potassium
- A third more magnesium
- Vitamin B6 and niacin

You probably know that physical exercise burns calories, but it can also help your weight loss efforts in other ways. Exercise is a good way to spend free time that prevents mindless snacking, exercise is a better way of dealing with negative emotions than eating, and moderate exercise can actually help to curb your appetite.

While there are plenty of exercise equipment options to help you get fit in your living room while you watch TV, these are not necessary. If you like the idea of watching your favorite show while you work out, consider a couple pairs of dumbbells in different weights.

When the weather is nice, however, consider getting a little extra Vitamin D and family time by getting your spouse and kids to join you for a walk.

The more you exercise, the more it gets to be a habit and you may find your day is incomplete if you aren't able to fit it in.

Work Out to Manage Stress

Overeating is a common coping mechanism to deal with daily pressure. When you find yourself craving a snack, try going for a walk instead. Exercise is a natural stress reliever.

Your body responds to stress by flooding your bloodstream with hormones such as adrenaline and cortisol. In a life threatening situation, these hormones are important to giving you the ability to manage the threat, either by running or fighting. However, your body doesn't know the difference between being behind at work or facing down a tiger, it releases the same hormones either way.

Today, most of the stressors we encounter don't give us the opportunity to burn off these hormones, so they build up. These hormones can interfere with sleep and impair your immune system.

What most people don't realize is that, not only does exercise help you burn off these hormones, but that a lack of exercise is actually a stressor of its own. Without exercise, you lose strength, flexibility, and muscle tone, as well as adding pounds.

Boost Your Mood

Exercise releases endorphins that can raise your mood and relieve pain. It can also improve your concentration, and studies have shown exercise to be an effective treatment for depression.

Exercise Can Be Easy

At work, you can go for a walk, climb stairs, or stretch at your desk. At home, your options increase. You can garden, most the lawn, or play with the kids. When shopping, walk an extra lap, or ride your bike to get there. Whatever you do, if you make it something you enjoy, it will be easier to stick with.

While exercise curbs your appetite for a time, your body will eventually want to replenish some of the calories burned. However, when you get hungry after exercising, it's real hunger and you're more likely to reach for nourishing fare.

Instructions:

Start slow, and perform the exercises without discomfort. Once you are used to the movements, try to complete the recommended sets and repetitions, taking 90 to 120 second break between exercises.

Workout Plan

Week	Monday	Wednesday	Friday
Week 1	Workout #1 + Stretching	Workout #1 + Stretching	Workout #1 + Stretching
Week 2	Workout #2 + Stretching	Workout #2 + Stretching	Workout #2 + Stretching
Week 3	Workout #3 + Stretching	Workout #3 + Stretching	Workout #3 + Stretching
Other Weeks	Workout #1 + Stretching	Workout #2 + Stretching	Workout #3 + Stretching

Exercise	Reps.	Sets	Rest
Forward Leg Hip Swings	10	1	120 secs
Side Leg / Hip Swings	10	1	120 secs
Chair Squat	10	2	120 secs
Knee Push-up	10	2	120 secs
Bodyweight Walking Lunge	10	2	120 secs
Superman / Extended Arms & Legs ✗ Lift	10	2	120 secs
Bird Dogs / Alternating Reach & ✗ Kickback	6	2	120 secs
- Dead Bug	10	2	120 secs
Hip Raise / Butt Lift / Bridge	15	1	120 secs

✗ on stomach raise hands & legs at same time
- on all fours, left leg up, right arm up
- lay on back, raise knees & arms
  extend one leg down, arm over head
- on back, arms on side lift hip

Exercise	Reps.	Sets	Rest
Donkey Kicks	10 *all 4's bent knees, kick up*	3	120 secs
Fire Hydrants / Abductor Knee Raise	10 *4's, knee bend up to side*	3	120 secs
Hip Raise / Butt Lift / Bridge	10 *on back - raise hips*	3	120 secs
Wall Sit / Squat / Chair	15 secs.	3	120 secs
Push-up	10	3	120 secs
Mountain Climbers / Alternating Knee-ins	*on 4's8, knees up to chest*	3	120 secs
Lying Leg Raise / Lift	15 *on back, hands under butt*	2	*raise legs* 120 secs
Leg Pull-In Knee-up	12	2	120 secs

- *sit hands behind butt, knees bent and up - reverse using hands reaching out*

Exercise	Reps.	Sets	Rest
Knee Push-up	10	3	120 secs
Cross Body Mountain ✗ Climbers	12	3	120 secs
Chair Squat	10	3	120 secs
Wall Sit / Squat / Chair	10 secs.	3	120 secs
Superman / Extended Arms & Legs Lift	12	3	120 secs
Single Leg Gluten Bridge / Hip Extension	8	3	120 secs
Side Plank	10	2	120 secs
Sit-ups	15	2	120 secs
Jumping Jacks / Star Jumps	10	1	120 secs

✗ 4's - knee up to opposite hand
- lay on back, one leg bent on heel, extend other then lift, butt up.

Building Resilience to Manage Stress

Resilience refers to how easily you recover from setbacks. There are a variety of factors that influence how you handle stress, but you can increase your resilience by learning coping mechanisms and by viewing situations differently. In doing so, you will find yourself less likely to overeat. Here are some ways to increase your resilience:

- Believe in yourself – Resilient people are confident. Believing in yourself will help you to deal with people who would seek to hurt you. Build your confidence by venturing beyond your comfort zone. Join a club or church, take up a hobby, or participate in other activities. Seek out people with whom you have things in common.
- Look on the bright side – People who see the good in less than ideal situations live longer, healthier lives than pessimists. Find the good in difficulties, and you'll feel better.
- Friendships – Cultivating supportive relationships gives you people to call on when you are down and give you a feeling of belonging. That said, don't allow anyone to take advantage of you. Learning to stand up to people you are close to without hurting feelings gives you practice that makes it easier to stand up to other diplomatically.
- Enjoy life – Be sure to set aside time every day to do something you like to do, whether that be a sport, craft, or other pastime.
- Laugh – Laughter truly is the best medicine. Studies have shown that people who have a good belly laugh every day experience less pain and depression than those who don't.
- Learn – Learning something new every day makes it easier to adjust to new situations and keeps your brain healthy and young. Seek out extra training and new responsibilities at

work, or learn a new skill at home.

- Listen to your gut – If you haven't paid much attention to your intuition lately, you may think you are lacking in that area. Practice listening to that little voice in the back of your mind. It may not be perfect, but is more reliable than many other ways of making decisions.
- Persevere – Set goals and do what it takes to achieve them. Failure is only permanent if you stop trying. If you have trouble following through, try setting some easy goals and seeing them through.
- Communicate – Resolve issues with open and honest communication and find a resolution that doesn't compromise your values.
- Take care of yourself – When you take good care of yourself, you feel better about yourself, which makes it easier for you to manage your stress. Be sure to eat a nutritious diet that includes plenty of fruits and vegetables, lean meats, and whole grains. Alcohol and caffeine are drugs, limit how much you consume. Exercise regularly and meditate or practice relaxation techniques.

Sample Meal Plan for a Day

Breakfast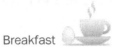

Recipe	Avg. Calories	Ready in
Breakfast Recipe	200	<20 Min.
Detox Smoothie	150	5 Min.

Lunch

Recipe	Avg. Calories	Ready in
Sugar-Blocking Salad	50	5 Min.
Lunch Recipe	200	<20 Min.
Fruits or Nuts	150	

Snack

Recipe	Avg. Calories	Ready in
Snack Recipe	100	5 Min.

Dinner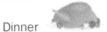

Recipe	Avg. Calories	Ready in
Sugar-Blocking Salad	50	5 Min.
Dinner Recipe	200	<25 Min.
Dessert	100	5 Min.

Sugar Blocking Salad Dressing

Consuming Vinegar before a meal containing carbs may lower blood sugar spikes. Simply eat this salad with a vinegar-based dressing for lunch or dinner.

This is much more effective (and easy) than cutting massively on carbs. Fill your salad dressing container with these ingredients and shake to combine all ingredients well:

1/3 container with balsamic wine vinegar

1/3 container with apple cider vinegar

1/3 container with (EVOO) extra virgin olive oil

Add a couple of Tsp. of real maple syrup

Add a touch of dried onion and garlic, and black pepper

Side Dish Salad

The following foods can be finely grated, chopped, or minced and mixed together:

1-2 Tomato

1-2 Carrot

1-2 Cup(s) Spinach or Lettuce

Breakfast Recipes

Greek Yoghurt and Fruit Salad

🍽 Makes: 2 🕐 Ready in: 10 min 🍴 Meal: Breakfast

Ingredients & Directions:

8 oz Greek yogurt

2 tbsp fresh fruit salad

4 tbsp raw honey

Alternately layer fruit salad and yogurt in a glass.

Drizzle honey over the top.

If you wish, you can sprinkle a few chopped walnuts and a bit of cinnamon on top.

Nutritional Facts x 1 Serving(s):

- Calories: 165
- Fat: 9 g
- Sat. Fat: 0 g
- Cholesterol: 0 mg
- Carbs: 19 g
- Sugars (Naturally-Occurring): 17 g
- Fiber: 1 g
- Protein: 2 g
- Sodium: 1 mg

Diet Tags:

- 🌳 Gluten:
- 🥛 Dairy:
- Acidic: Yes
- Low Sodium: Yes
- Low Cholesterol: Yes
- Low Carb: Yes
- Diabetics: Yes

Buckwheat

Ingredients & Directions:

2 cups water

1/4 tsp salt

1 cup Kasha

Bring the water to a boil in a medium pan.

Add salt and buckwheat to the boiling water.

Reduce heat, cover, and simmer about ten minutes, or until all water is absorbed.

Nutritional Facts x 1 Serving(s):

- Calories: 108
- Fat: 0 g
- Sat. Fat: 0 g
- Cholesterol: 0 mg
- Carbs: 24 g
- Sugars (Naturally-Occurring): 1 g
- Fiber: 3 g
- Protein: 3 g
- Sodium: 122 mg

Diet Tags:

- Gluten:
- Dairy:
- Acidic:
- Low Sodium: Yes
- Low Cholesterol: Yes
- Low Carb: Yes
- Diabetics: Yes

Delicious Oatmeal

⏏ Makes: 2 🕐 Ready in: 16 min 🍴 Meal: Breakfast

👨‍🍳 Ingredients & Directions:

1/2 cup Rolled Oats (Certified gluten-free if you are gluten intolerant)

1 cup low-fat milk (or soy/almond milk)

1 cup Frozen Berries

Combine oats and milk in a medium saucepan.

Bring to a boil, reduce heat and simmer, stirring occasionally until thickened.

Add berries and continue cooking until the berries are warm.

Nutritional Facts x 1 Serving(s):

- Calories: 109
- Fat: 1 g
- Sat. Fat: 0 g
- Cholesterol: 2 mg
- Carbs: 19 g
- Sugars (Naturally-Occurring): 6 g
- Fiber: 2 g
- Protein: 6 g
- Sodium: 52 mg

Diet Tags:

- 🌳 Gluten:
- 🥛 Dairy:
- 🔥 Acidic:
- Low Sodium: Yes
- 💚 Low Cholesterol: Yes
- Low Carb: Yes
- Diabetics: Yes

Fat Free Pancake

🛎 Makes: 1.0 🕐 Ready in: 7 min 🍴 Meal: Breakfast

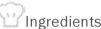Ingredients & Directions:

1/4 cup Whole Wheat Flour (gluten-free alternative: brown rice flour or certified gluten-free oat flour)

1 pinch baking soda

1 pinch salt

1 drop vanilla extract

Skim or nondairy milk, to taste

Mix all ingredients thoroughly in a bowl.

Coat a pan with Extra Virgin Olive Oil.

Pour batter into hot pan.

Cook over medium heat. Flip when edges bubble.

Nutritional Facts x 1 Serving(s):

- Calories: 96
- Fat: 0 g
- Sat. Fat: 0 g
- Cholesterol: 0 mg
- Carbs: 21 g
- Sugars (Naturally-Occurring): 0 g
- Fiber: 3 g
- Protein: 3 g
- Sodium: 219 mg

Diet Tags:

- 🌳 Gluten:
- 🥛 Dairy:
- Acidic:
- Low Sodium: Yes
- 💚 Low Cholesterol: Yes
- Low Carb: Yes
- Diabetics: Yes

Egg White Scramble

 Makes: 1 🕐 Ready in: 10 min 🍴 Meal: Breakfast

Ingredients & Directions:

3 egg whites

1/4 cup chopped tomatoes

1/4 cup diced onions

1/4 cup diced peppers

1/4 cup sliced jalapenos (not required)

Sauté all ingredients except egg whites in a non-stick pan until onions begin to soften.

Add eggs and scramble all ingredients together.

Salt and pepper to taste.

Nutritional Facts x 1 Serving(s):

- Calories: 157
- Fat: 1 g
- Sat. Fat: 0 g
- Cholesterol: 0 mg
- Carbs: 23 g
- Sugars (Naturally-Occurring): 3 g
- Fiber: 8 g
- Protein: 14 g
- Sodium: 179 mg

Diet Tags:

- 🌳 Gluten:
- 🥛 Dairy:
- 🔥 Acidic: Yes
- 🧂 Low Sodium: Yes
- ♥ Low Cholesterol: Yes
- Low Carb: Yes
- Diabetics: Yes

Unsweetened Applesauce-Cranberry Oatmeal

🍽 Makes: 1 🕐 Ready in: 4 min 🍴 Meal: Breakfast

👨‍🍳 Ingredients & Directions:

3 tbsp Oatmeal (Certified gluten-free if you are gluten intolerant), uncooked

1 tbsp dried cranberries

1/2 cup Unsweetened Applesauce

1/2 cup water

1/8 tsp ground cinnamon

Combine all ingredients in a bowl and microwave 1-2 minutes.

🍎 Nutritional Facts x 1 Serving(s):

- Calories: 113
- Fat: 1 g
- Sat. Fat: 0 g
- Cholesterol: 0 mg
- Carbs: 24 g
- Sugars (Naturally-Occurring): 11 g
- Fiber: 3 g
- Protein: 2 g
- Sodium: 7 mg

🍴 Diet Tags:

- 🌳 Gluten:
- 🥛 Dairy:
- Acidic: Yes
- Low Sodium: Yes
- 💚 Low Cholesterol: Yes
- Low Carb: Yes
- Diabetics: Yes

3-Ingredient Cinnamon Banana Slice

 Makes: 1.0 ⏱ Ready in: 5 min 🍴 Meal: Breakfast

Ingredients & Directions:

1 slice 100% Whole Grain Bread
(Gluten-Free Alternative: Brown Rice
Bread)

1/2 small banana, sliced

pinch of cinnamon

Preheat nonstick griddle.

Heat bread on griddle for one
minute.

Cover bread with banana slices and
sprinkle with cinnamon.

Press the bread gently with a
spatula.

Remove when the bottom of the
bread turns golden brown.

🍎 Nutritional Facts x 1 Serving(s):

- Calories: 117
- Fat: 1 g
- Sat. Fat: 0 g
- Cholesterol: 0 mg
- Carbs: 24 g
- Sugars (Naturally-Occurring): 7 g
- Fiber: 3 g
- Protein: 3 g
- Sodium: 148 mg

Diet Tags:

- 🌴 Gluten:
- 🥛 Dairy:
- Acidic:
- 🧂 Low Sodium: Yes
- ♥ Low Cholesterol: Yes
- Low Carb: Yes
- Diabetics: Yes

Natural Peanut Butter Oatmeal

⌂ Makes: 1 🕐 Ready in: 5 min 🍴 Meal: Breakfast

 Ingredients & Directions:

1/4 cup Rolled Oats (Certified gluten-free if you are gluten intolerant)

1/2 cup nonfat milk (or soy/almond milk)

1 tbsp Natural Peanut Butter

1/4 tsp ground cinnamon

Combine oats and milk in a microwave safe bowl and microwave on high 3 minutes.

Add peanut butter and cinnamon and stir well. Add more milk as desired to taste.

 Nutritional Facts x 1 Serving(s):

- Calories: 213
- Fat: 9 g
- Sat. Fat: 1 g
- Cholesterol: 2 mg
- Carbs: 23 g
- Sugars (Naturally-Occurring): 7 g
- Fiber: 3 g
- Protein: 10 g
- Sodium: 126 mg

 Diet Tags:

- 🌳 Gluten:
- 🥛 Dairy:
- 🔥 Acidic:
- Low Sodium: Yes
- 💙 Low Cholesterol: Yes
- Low Carb: Yes
- Diabetics: Yes

Stuffed Apples

 Makes: 2 Ready in: 5 min Meal: Breakfast

Ingredients & Directions:

1 apple , of your choice

1/4 cup corn flakes ✓

6 tsp Natural Peanut Butter

Core apple and cut apple in half.

Use a spoon to scoop out apple to about ¼ inch of the peel.

Mix apple, corn flakes, and peanut butter well in a bowl.

Scoop the mix back into the apple shells.

Nutritional Facts x 1 Serving(s):

- Calories: 152
- Fat: 8 g
- Sat. Fat: 1 g
- Cholesterol: 0 mg
- Carbs: 16 g
- Sugars (Naturally-Occurring): 8 g
- Fiber: 3 g
- Protein: 4 g
- Sodium: 103 mg

Diet Tags:

- Gluten:
- Dairy:
- Acidic:
- Low Sodium: Yes
- Low Cholesterol: Yes
- Low Carb: Yes
- Diabetics: Yes

Detox Smoothies

Strawberry Flax Smoothie

🍽 Makes: Serves 2. 1 cup per serving. 🕐 Ready in: 5 min 🍴 Meal: Breakfast

Ingredients & Directions:

1 cup fresh or defrosted frozen sliced strawberries

1/2 cup Fat Free Vanilla Yogurt

1/2 cup Low-Fat Milk (or soy/almond milk)

3 tbsp Ground Flaxseed

1/2 tsp ground cinnamon

Combine all ingredients in a blender on high until smooth.

Pour into a glass. May be served immediately or refrigerated for up to 2 hours.

Nutritional Facts x 1 Serving(s):

- Calories: 141
- Fat: 5 g
- Sat. Fat: 0 g
- Cholesterol: 3 mg
- Carbs: 18 g
- Sugars (Naturally-Occurring): 10 g
- Fiber: 4 g
- Protein: 6 g
- Sodium: 66 mg

Diet Tags:

- 🌳 Gluten:
- 🥛 Dairy:
- Acidic:
- Low Sodium: Yes
- Low Cholesterol: Yes
- Low Carb: Yes
- Diabetics: Yes

Spinach Banana Smoothie

 Makes: 2 🕐 Ready in: 5 min 🍴 Meal: Breakfast

Ingredients & Directions:

4 cups baby spinach, raw

6 oz vanilla yogurt , 1 serving

1 banana

Put all ingredients in blender and blend on high 1-2 minutes. If too thick, add water a little at a time and blend to thin.

🍎 Nutritional Facts x 1 Serving(s):

- Calories: 123
- Fat: 3 g
- Sat. Fat: 1 g
- Cholesterol: 11 mg
- Carbs: 19 g
- Sugars (Naturally-Occurring): 11 g
- Fiber: 2 g
- Protein: 5 g
- Sodium: 87 mg

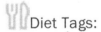Diet Tags:

- 🌳 Gluten:
- 🥛 Dairy:
- 🔥 Acidic:
- 🧂 Low Sodium: Yes
- ♥ Low Cholesterol: Yes
- ▼ Low Carb: Yes
- ○ Diabetics: Yes

Simple Smoothies

△ Makes: 1 ◷ Ready in: 7 min 🍴 Meal: Breakfast

Ingredients & Directions:

1/2 Cup of Frozen Berries

1/4 Cup of Frozen Strawberries

1 Cup of Fat Free Vanilla Yogurt

4 Ice Cubes

Water

Place all ingredients in a blender and blend until smooth.

Nutritional Facts x 1 Serving(s):

- Calories: 116
- Fat: 0 g
- Sat. Fat: 0 g
- Cholesterol: 0 mg
- Carbs: 24 g
- Sugars (Naturally-Occurring): 1 g
- Fiber: 3 g
- Protein: 5 g
- Sodium: 81 mg

Diet Tags:

- 🌳 Gluten:
- 🥛 Dairy:
- 🌶 Acidic:
- Low Sodium: Yes
- Low Cholesterol: Yes
- Low Carb: Yes
- Diabetics: Yes

Honeydew Smoothies

Makes: 2 🕐 Ready in: 5 min 🍴 Meal: Breakfast

👨‍🍳 Ingredients & Directions:

2 cups honeydew melon , cubed

1/2 cup vanilla yogurt

1/4 tsp vanilla extract

1 cup ice

Place all ingredients in a blender and blend until frothy.

🍎 Nutritional Facts x 1 Serving(s):

- Calories: 106
- Fat: 2 g
- Sat. Fat: 1 g
- Cholesterol: 7 mg
- Carbs: 19 g
- Sugars (Naturally-Occurring): 17 g
- Fiber: 1 g
- Protein: 3 g
- Sodium: 63 mg

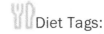 Diet Tags:

- 🌳 Gluten:
- 🥛 Dairy:
- 🔥 Acidic:
- Low Sodium: Yes
- 💚 Low Cholesterol: Yes
- Low Carb: Yes
- Diabetics: Yes

OJ & Strawberry Smoothie

Makes: 1 ⏲ Ready in: 10 min 🍴 Meal: Breakfast

Ingredients & Directions:

1/2 Cup Orange Juice
(Unsweetened)

1 cup fresh strawberries

1 berry flavored yogurt

5 ice cubes

Place all ingredients in a blender
and blend until smooth.

Nutritional Facts x 1 Serving(s):

- Calories: 92
- Fat: 0 g
- Sat. Fat: 0 g
- Cholesterol: 0 mg
- Carbs: 22 g
- Sugars (Naturally-Occurring): 1 g
- Fiber: 3 g
- Protein: 1 g
- Sodium: 2 mg

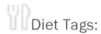 Diet Tags:

- 🌳 Gluten:
- 🥛 Dairy:
- Acidic: Yes
- Low Sodium: Yes
- Low Cholesterol: Yes
- Low Carb: Yes
- Diabetics: Yes

Delicious Dairy Free Smoothie

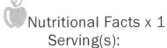 Makes: 2 Ready in: 5 min Meal: Breakfast

Ingredients & Directions:

1 1/2 cups Soymilk (Unsweetened) , vanilla

1/2-3/4 cup frozen berries

1 tsp honey

Place all ingredients in a blender and blend until smooth.

Nutritional Facts x 1 Serving(s):

- Calories: 103
- Fat: 3 g
- Sat. Fat: 0 g
- Cholesterol: 0 mg
- Carbs: 14 g
- Sugars (Naturally-Occurring): 10 g
- Fiber: 1 g
- Protein: 5 g
- Sodium: 93 mg

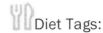Diet Tags:

- Gluten:
- Dairy:
- Acidic:
- Low Sodium: Yes
- Low Cholesterol: Yes
- Low Carb: Yes
- Diabetics: Yes

Banana Shake

Ingredients & Directions:

1 1/2 cups Low-Fat Milk (or soy/almond milk)

1 frozen banana

1/2 tsp vanilla extract

1/4 tsp almond extract

Place all ingredients in a blender and blend until smooth.

Nutritional Facts x 1 Serving(s):

- Calories: 120
- Fat: 0 g
- Sat. Fat: 0 g
- Cholesterol: 3 mg
- Carbs: 23 g
- Sugars (Naturally-Occurring): 7 g
- Fiber: 1 g
- Protein: 7 g
- Sodium: 109 mg

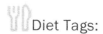Diet Tags:

- 🌳 Gluten:
- 🥛 Dairy:
- 🔥 Acidic: Yes
- 🧂 Low Sodium: Yes
- 💚 Low Cholesterol: Yes
- 🍴 Low Carb: Yes
- ○ Diabetics: Yes

Cucumber, Apple, and Mint Cooler

 Makes: 2 srv (serving size: 1 cup) ⏱ Ready in: 20 min 🍴 Meal: Breakfast

👨‍🍳 Ingredients & Directions:

1 cup chopped cucumber

1/3 cup Frozen, 100% Apple Juice Concentrate

1/4 cup cold water

1/4 cup chopped fresh mint

10 ice cubes

Place all ingredients in a blender and blend until smooth.

Nutritional Facts x 1 Serving(s):

- Calories: 88
- Fat: 0 g
- Sat. Fat: 0 g
- Cholesterol: 0 mg
- Carbs: 21 g
- Sugars (Naturally-Occurring): 1 g
- Fiber: 1 g
- Protein: 1 g
- Sodium: 16 mg

Diet Tags:

- 🌳 Gluten:
- 🥛 Dairy:
- 🔥 Acidic: Yes
- Low Sodium: Yes
- ♥ Low Cholesterol: Yes
- Low Carb: Yes
- Diabetics: Yes

Cocoa Banana Smoothie

🛎 Makes: 4 🕐 Ready in: 6 min 🍴 Meal: Breakfast

👨‍🍳 Ingredients & Directions:

2 tbsp Unsweetened Cocoa Powder

7 oz Cream of Coconut

2 cups Low-Fat Milk (or soy/almond milk)

2 frozen bananas , peeled

Place all ingredients in a blender and blend until smooth.

Best served immediately.

Nutritional Facts x 1 Serving(s):

- Calories: 108
- Fat: 0 g
- Sat. Fat: 0 g
- Cholesterol: 2 mg
- Carbs: 21 g
- Sugars (Naturally-Occurring): 7 g
- Fiber: 2 g
- Protein: 6 g
- Sodium: 73 mg

Diet Tags:

- 🌳 Gluten:
- 🥛 Dairy:
- 🔥 Acidic: Yes
- 🧂 Low Sodium: Yes
- 💗 Low Cholesterol: Yes
- Low Carb: Yes
- Diabetics: Yes

Ginger Berry Zing

 Makes: 2 ⏱ Ready in: 5 min 🍴 Meal: Breakfast

Ingredients & Directions:

1 1/2 cups water , to taste

1 large banana

1 cup berries , frozen

1 tbsp fresh ginger

1/8 cup Flaxseed , ground

Place all ingredients in a blender and blend until smooth.

Serves 2

Nutritional Facts x 1 Serving(s):

- Calories: 120
- Fat: 4 g
- Sat. Fat: 0 g
- Cholesterol: 0 mg
- Carbs: 19 g
- Sugars (Naturally-Occurring): 8 g
- Fiber: 4 g
- Protein: 2 g
- Sodium: 7 mg

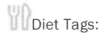 Diet Tags:

- 🌳 Gluten:
- 🥛 Dairy:
- Acidic:
- Low Sodium: Yes
- Low Cholesterol: Yes
- Low Carb: Yes
- Diabetics: Yes

Sunrise Smoothie

🍽 Makes: 1 🕐 Ready in: 10 min 🍴 Meal: Breakfast

 Ingredients & Directions:

3/4 cup Fat Free Vanilla Yogurt

1 cup strawberry , fresh, frozen (or any other berry)

1/4 cup Orange Juice (Unsweetened)

2 ice cubes

1 tbsp Ground Flaxseed

Crush ice in blender.

Add fresh or frozen berries and blend.

Add the remainder of ingredients and blend once more until smooth. Add unsweetened orange juice if the result is too thick.

 Nutritional Facts x 1 Serving(s):

- Calories: 111
- Fat: 3 g
- Sat. Fat: 0 g
- Cholesterol: 0 mg
- Carbs: 19 g
- Sugars (Naturally-Occurring): 12 g
- Fiber: 4 g
- Protein: 2 g
- Sodium: 5 mg

 Diet Tags:

- 🌳 Gluten:
- 🥛 Dairy:
- 🔥 Acidic: Yes
- Low Sodium: Yes
- Low Cholesterol: Yes
- Low Carb: Yes
- Diabetics: Yes

Strawberry Mango

🍽 Makes: 3 - 1/2 cup 🕐 Ready in: 5 min 🍴 Meal: Breakfast

Ingredients & Directions:

2 frozen bananas ✓

1/2 cup frozen strawberries

1/2 frozen mango, peeled and cut in strips

Directions:

Run all ingredients through a food processor.

Nutritional Facts x 1 Serving(s):

- Calories: 125
- Fat: 1 g
- Sat. Fat: 0 g
- Cholesterol: 0 mg
- Carbs: 28 g
- Sugars (Naturally-Occurring): 19 g
- Fiber: 3 g
- Protein: 1 g
- Sodium: 2 mg

Diet Tags:

- 🌳 Gluten:
- 🥛 Dairy:
- 🍋 Acidic:
- Low Sodium: Yes
- 💙 Low Cholesterol: Yes
- Low Carb: Yes
- Diabetics: Yes

Pumpkin Spice Smoothie

🍽 Makes: 1 🕐 Ready in: 4 min 🍴 Meal: Snack

👨‍🍳 Ingredients & Directions:

½ can pumpkin puree

½ cup low-fat plain kefir

¼ cup orange juice

1 tsp agave nectar

1/8 tsp pumpkin pie spice

1/3 cup crushed ice

Blend all ingredients until smooth.

Nutritional Facts x 1 Serving(s):

- Calories: 130
- Fat: 2 g
- Sat. Fat: 0 g
- Cholesterol: 4 mg
- Carbs: 23 g
- Sugars (Naturally-Occurring): 1 g
- Fiber: 4 g
- Protein: 5 g
- Sodium: 125 mg

Diet Tags:

- 🌳Gluten:
- 🥛Dairy:
- 🔥Acidic:
- 🧂Low Sodium: Yes
- 💗Low Cholesterol: Yes
- Low Carb: Yes
- Diabetics: Yes

Lunch

Garlic Squash Chicken

Makes: 1 ⏱ Ready in: 15 min 🍴 Meal: Lunch

Ingredients & Directions:

Summer squash, 1 cup, chopped

Chicken Breast (Boneless Skinless), 1 oz

1 tsp each Onion powder and garlic powder

Extra Virgin Olive Oil, 1 1tsp

Cut squash and chicken each into 1 inch cubes.

Put Extra Virgin Olive Oil into a preheated pan and add chicken, onion powder, and garlic powder.

Cook for 1-2 minutes, then add squash and cook until chicken is thoroughly cooked.

Nutritional Facts x 1 Serving(s):

- Calories: 105
- Fat: 5 g
- Sat. Fat: 0 g
- Cholesterol: 16 mg
- Carbs: 7 g
- Sugars (Naturally-Occurring): 0 g
- Fiber: 1 g
- Protein: 8 g
- Sodium: 24 mg

Diet Tags:

- 🌳 Gluten:
- 🥛 Dairy:
- Acidic: Yes
- Low Sodium: Yes
- Low Cholesterol: Yes
- Low Carb: Yes
- Diabetics: Yes

Cashew Chicken Salad

🔔 Makes: 6 srv (serving size: 1/2 cup) 🕐 Ready in: 20 min 🍴 Meal: Lunch

👨‍🍳 Ingredients & Directions:

1/4 cup Fat Free vanilla Yogurt

3 tbsp Light Mayonnaise

1/4 tsp curry powder

2 cups shredded cooked Chicken Breast

1 cup sliced red seedless grapes

1/3 cup chopped celery

2 tbsp chopped salted dry-roasted cashews

1 tbsp finely chopped green onions

Combine yogurt, mayonnaise, and curry powder in a bowl.

Add remaining ingredients and stir well to ensure chicken is coated.

Cover and chill.

🍎 Nutritional Facts x 1 Serving(s):

- Calories: 137
- Fat: 5 g
- Sat. Fat: 1 g
- Cholesterol: 43 mg
- Carbs: 8 g
- Sugars (Naturally-Occurring): 0 g
- Fiber: 0 g
- Protein: 15 g
- Sodium: 125 mg

🍴 Diet Tags:

- 🌳 Gluten:
- 🥛 Dairy:
- Acidic: Yes
- 🧂 Low Sodium: Yes
- 💙 Low Cholesterol: Yes
- Low Carb: Yes
- Diabetics: Yes

Easy and Delicious Chicken Salad

 Makes: 2 ⏲ Ready in: 5 min 🍴 Meal: Lunch

Ingredients & Directions:

1 cup cooked Chicken Meat, diced or shredded (grill, broil, steam or use a rotisserie chicken)

2 tbsp Light Mayonnaise

1/4 cup crunchy grapes , quartered (red or green)

1/4 tsp sea salt

Combine all ingredients and chill. Serve cold.

Nutritional Facts x 1 Serving(s):

- Calories: 114
- Fat: 2 g
- Sat. Fat: 0 g
- Cholesterol: 59 mg
- Carbs: 3 g
- Sugars (Naturally-Occurring): 2 g
- Fiber: 0 g
- Protein: 21 g
- Sodium: 342 mg

Diet Tags:

- 🌳 Gluten:
- 🥛 Dairy:
- 🍋 Acidic:
- 🧺 Low Sodium: Yes
- 💙 Low Cholesterol: Yes
- Low Carb: Yes
- Diabetics: Yes

Hummus Wrap with Tomatoes and Spinach

🛎 Makes: 2 🕐 Ready in: 5 min 🍴 Meal: Lunch

Ingredients & Directions:

2 Flour Tortillas (Gluten-Free alternative: Yellow Corn Tortillas)

1/4 cup hummus

1/4 cup chopped tomato

1/4 cup fresh spinach , shredded

1 tsp Extra Virgin Olive Oil

Spread 2 Tbsp hummus on each wrap.

Top each wrap with 1/8 cup each of tomato and spinach.

Drizzle with Extra Virgin Olive Oil.

Add onion (optional) and fold wrap.

Nutritional Facts x 1 Serving(s):

- Calories: 145
- Fat: 5 g
- Sat. Fat: 1 g
- Cholesterol: 0 mg
- Carbs: 20 g
- Sugars (Naturally-Occurring): 1 g
- Fiber: 3 g
- Protein: 5 g
- Sodium: 311 mg

Diet Tags:

- Gluten:
- Dairy:
- Acidic: Yes
- Low Sodium: Yes
- Low Cholesterol: Yes
- Low Carb: Yes
- Diabetics: Yes

Egg White Avocado Salad

🔔 Makes: 4 srv 🕐 Ready in: 5 min 🍴 Meal: Lunch

Ingredients & Directions:

6 large egg whites, boiled and chopped

2 tbsps Light Mayonnaise

1 medium granny smith apple

1 avocado, chopped

1 fl oz lemon juice

1/2 cup shredded or chopped lettuce

1 tbsp parsley, minced

Arrange lettuce on a plate.

Toss all other ingredients gently in a bowl and place on lettuce bed.

🍎 Nutritional Facts x 1 Serving(s):

- Calories: 154
- Fat: 10 g
- Sat. Fat: 1 g
- Cholesterol: 3 mg
- Carbs: 10 g
- Sugars (Naturally-Occurring): 4 g
- Fiber: 3 g
- Protein: 6 g
- Sodium: 137 mg

Diet Tags:

- 🌳 Gluten:
- 🥛 Dairy:
- Acidic: Yes
- 🧂 Low Sodium: Yes
- 💙 Low Cholesterol: Yes
- Low Carb: Yes
- ⭕ Diabetics: Yes

Apple Broccoli Waldorf

🍲 Makes: 4- 1 cup per serving 🕐 Ready in: 5 min 🍴 Meal: Lunch

👨‍🍳 Ingredients & Directions:

2 red apples, diced

2 cups broccoli flowers

2 tbsp chopped green onion

2 tbsp chopped walnuts

1/4 cup raisins

1/2 cup low-fat vanilla yogurt

Mix all ingredients and chill.

Serve cold on a bed of lettuce

🍎 Nutritional Facts x 1 Serving(s):

- Calories: 139
- Fat: 3 g
- Sat. Fat: 0 g
- Cholesterol: 0 mg
- Carbs: 24 g
- Sugars (Naturally-Occurring): 19 g
- Fiber: 3 g
- Protein: 4 g
- Sodium: 35 mg

Diet Tags:

- 🌾 Gluten:
- 🥛 Dairy:
- 🍋 Acidic: Yes
- 🧂 Low Sodium: Yes
- ♥ Low Cholesterol: Yes
- 🌿 Low Carb: Yes
- ○ Diabetics: Yes

Garbanzo and Rice Salad

🔔 Makes: 10 srv 🕐 Ready in: 10 min 🍽 Meal: Lunch

Ingredients & Directions: ✓

1/2 tsp dill

4 tbsps red wine vinegar

1/2 cup chopped red onion

2 cups chopped green pepper

1 cup chopped or sliced tomato

2 cups garbanzo beans

2 cups cooked brown rice

Combine all ingredients in a bowl and toss.

Nutritional Facts x 1 Serving(s):

- Calories: 104
- Fat: 0 g
- Sat. Fat: 0 g
- Cholesterol: 0 mg
- Carbs: 23 g
- Sugars (Naturally-Occurring): 1 g
- Fiber: 3 g
- Protein: 3 g
- Sodium: 146 mg

Diet Tags:

- 🌳 Gluten:
- 🥛 Dairy:
- Acidic: Yes
- Low Sodium: Yes
- Low Cholesterol: Yes
- Low Carb: Yes
- Diabetics: Yes

Sloppy Joes

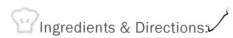 Makes: 8 Ready in: 20 min Meal: Lunch

Ingredients & Directions:

1 Lb Lean ground turkey

1 Package sloppy joe mix

1 can (6oz) Tomato Paste (No-Salt-Added)

1 1/4 cups water

Brown turkey over medium heat and drain fat.

Add seasoning mix, tomato paste, and water, stirring well.

Heat to a boil, then lower heat.

Simmer ten minutes, stirring occasionally.

Serve on whole grain hamburger bun.

Nutritional Facts x 1 Serving(s):

- Calories: 136
- Fat: 8 g
- Sat. Fat: 0 g
- Cholesterol: 42 mg
- Carbs: 6 g
- Sugars (Naturally-Occurring): 0 g
- Fiber: 1 g
- Protein: 10 g
- Sodium: 403 mg

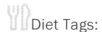 Diet Tags:

- Gluten:
- Dairy:
- Acidic: Yes
- Low Sodium: Yes
- Low Cholesterol: Yes
- Low Carb: Yes
- Diabetics: Yes

Papaya-Avocado Salad

🍽 Makes: 4 srv, about 2/3 cup each ⏱ Ready in: 10 min 🍴 Meal: Lunch

👨‍🍳 Ingredients & Directions:

1 medium papaya, diced

1 medium avocado, diced

3/4 cup diced jicama

2 tbsp chopped toasted walnuts

2 tbsp Light Raspberry Vinaigrette

Toss all ingredients gently in a bowl.

🍎 Nutritional Facts x 1 Serving(s):

- Calories: 124
- Fat: 8 g
- Sat. Fat: 1 g
- Cholesterol: 0 mg
- Carbs: 11 g
- Sugars (Naturally-Occurring): 0 g
- Fiber: 5 g
- Protein: 2 g
- Sodium: 25 mg

🍴 Diet Tags:

- 🌳 Gluten:
- 🥛 Dairy:
- 🔥 Acidic: Yes
- 🧂 Low Sodium: Yes
- 💟 Low Cholesterol: Yes
- 🌱 Low Carb: Yes
- ⏰ Diabetics: Yes

PB Toast

🛎 Makes: 1 🕐 Ready in: 5 min 🍴 Meal: Lunch

Ingredients & Directions: ✓

1 slice rye (preferred), whole wheat, or Brown Rice Bread

Natural Peanut Butter

Tomato slices

Salt and Pepper to taste

Toast bread

Spread peanut butter on toast while still hot.

Top with tomato slices

Spread Natural Peanut Butter on HOT toast.

Now, completely cover the toast with tomato slices. Cut slices as needed to completely cover toast.

Sprinkle with salt and pepper to taste. Serve hot.

Nutritional Facts x 1 Serving(s):

- Calories: 106
- Fat: 2 g
- Sat. Fat: 0 g
- Cholesterol: 20 mg
- Carbs: 19 g
- Sugars (Naturally-Occurring): 0 g
- Fiber: 0 g
- Protein: 3 g
- Sodium: 199 mg

Diet Tags:

- 🌳 Gluten:
- 🥛 Dairy:
- 🔥 Acidic:
- Low Sodium: Yes
- ♥ Low Cholesterol: Yes
- Low Carb: Yes
- ○ Diabetics: Yes

Yummy Zesty Zucchini Wrap

🍽 Makes: 2 🕐 Ready in: 20 min 🍴 Meal: Lunch

Ingredients & Directions: ✓

2 zucchini, green and yellow julienned

1 onion, diced

1 red bell pepper , julienned

2 tbsp Extra Virgin Olive Oil

1 cup baby spinach

1/2 cup guacamole

Heat pan with Extra Virgin Olive Oil. Saute' zucchini, bell pepper, and onion approximately ten minutes.

Add salt and pepper to taste. Spread guacamole on tortilla.

Add cooked veggies and the rest of the ingredients to the tortilla.

Wrap and serve hot or cold.

Nutritional Facts x 1 Serving(s):

- Calories: 202
- Fat: 14 g
- Sat. Fat: 2 g
- Cholesterol: 0 mg
- Carbs: 16 g
- Sugars (Naturally-Occurring): 8 g
- Fiber: 4 g
- Protein: 3 g
- Sodium: 34 mg

Diet Tags:

- 🌳 Gluten:
- 🥛 Dairy:
- Acidic: Yes
- Low Sodium: Yes
- Low Cholesterol: Yes
- Low Carb: Yes
- Diabetics: Yes

Mushroom Ceviche

🛎 Makes: 6 🕐 Ready in: 15 min 🍴 Meal: Lunch

Ingredients & Directions:

1 lb sliced fresh mushrooms

1 cup chopped red onion

2 cups tomatoes , diced

1 cup chopped cilantro

1 chopped habanero pepper (not required)

1/4 cup Extra Virgin Olive Oil

2 salt and pepper

Steam mushrooms until they just start to turn soft. Set aside to cool.

Add the rest of the ingredients.

Chill and serve with whole grain crackers, brown rice crackers, or tostadas.

Nutritional Facts x 1 Serving(s):

- Calories: 125
- Fat: 9 g
- Sat. Fat: 1 g
- Cholesterol: 0 mg
- Carbs: 8 g
- Sugars (Naturally-Occurring): 4 g
- Fiber: 2 g
- Protein: 3 g
- Sodium: 9 mg

Diet Tags:

- 🌳 Gluten:
- 🥛 Dairy:
- Acidic: Yes
- Low Sodium: Yes
- Low Cholesterol: Yes
- Low Carb: Yes
- Diabetics: Yes

TAO Sandwiches

🛎 Makes: 2 🕐 Ready in: 10 min 🍴 Meal: Lunch

👨‍🍳 Ingredients & Directions:

4 slices 100% Whole Grain Bread
(Gluten-Free Alternative: Brown Rice
Bread) (your choice)

1 large tomato, sliced

1 avocado, sliced

3 -5 slices red onions

1 dash Light Mayonnaise

Spread mayo on bread.

Arrange the rest of the ingredients.

Nutritional Facts x 1 Serving(s):

- Calories: 345
- Fat: 17 g
- Sat. Fat: 2 g
- Cholesterol: 0 mg
- Carbs: 40 g
- Sugars (Naturally-Occurring): 7 g
- Fiber: 11 g
- Protein: 8 g
- Sodium: 307 mg

🍴 Diet Tags:

- 🌳 Gluten:
- 🥛 Dairy:
- 💧 Acidic: Yes
- Low Sodium: Yes
- ♥ Low Cholesterol: Yes
- Low Carb:
- Diabetics: Yes

PB and Cucumber Sandwich

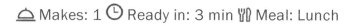

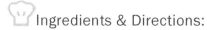Makes: 1 Ready in: 3 min Meal: Lunch

Ingredients & Directions:

2 slices 100% Whole Grain or Brown Rice Bread

Natural Peanut Butter

4 -5 slices of peeled cucumbers (thin slices)

Spread peanut butter on bread

Arrange cucumber.

Cover with the other slice of bread.

Nutritional Facts x 1 Serving(s):

- Calories: 129
- Fat: 1 g
- Sat. Fat: 0 g
- Cholesterol: 0 mg
- Carbs: 26 g
- Sugars (Naturally-Occurring): 2 g
- Fiber: 1 g
- Protein: 4 g
- Sodium: 341 mg

Diet Tags:

- Gluten:
- Dairy:
- Acidic:
- Low Sodium: Yes
- Low Cholesterol: Yes
- Low Carb:
- Diabetics: Yes

An Avocado-Licious Sandwich

🍽 Makes: 1 ⏱ Ready in: 5 min 🍴 Meal: Lunch

👨‍🍳 Ingredients & Directions:

2 slices 100% Whole Grain or Brown Rice Bread, toasted

1/2 small avocado, sliced

1/2 roma tomato, sliced

3 slices turkey breast

Start with one slice of bread.

Add turkey slice and tomato slices.

Sprinkle salt and pepper to taste.

Add avocado and second slice of bread.

Great with fresh melon!

Nutritional Facts x 1 Serving(s):

- Calories: 299
- Fat: 15 g
- Sat. Fat: 2 g
- Cholesterol: 0 mg
- Carbs: 34 g
- Sugars (Naturally-Occurring): 4 g
- Fiber: 10 g
- Protein: 7 g
- Sodium: 303 mg

Diet Tags:

- 🌳 Gluten:
- 🥛 Dairy:
- 🌶 Acidic: Yes
- 🧂 Low Sodium: Yes
- 💚 Low Cholesterol: Yes
- 🌱 Low Carb:
- ⭕ Diabetics: Yes

Avocado, Tomato, and Hummus Sandwich

🍽 Makes: 4.0 🕐 Ready in: 5 min 🍴 Meal: Lunch

Ingredients & Directions: ✓

1 medium tomato, sliced

1 medium avocado, cut in half and sliced long ways

4 tbsp hummus

8 slices 100% Whole Grain or Brown Rice Bread

Spread 1 Tbsp on each of 4 slices of bread.

Add 2 slices each of avocado and tomato to each slice.

Top with the rest of the bread.

Nutritional Facts x 1 Serving(s):

- Calories: 246
- Fat: 10 g
- Sat. Fat: 1 g
- Cholesterol: 0 mg
- Carbs: 30 g
- Sugars (Naturally-Occurring): 4 g
- Fiber: 8 g
- Protein: 9 g
- Sodium: 326 mg

Diet Tags:

- 🌳 Gluten:
- 🥛 Dairy:
- Acidic: Yes
- Low Sodium: Yes
- Low Cholesterol: Yes
- Low Carb:
- Diabetics: Yes

Chicken Avocado Sandwich

🍽 Makes: 1 🕐 Ready in: 10 min 🍴 Meal: Lunch

👨‍🍳 Ingredients & Directions:

1 tsp extra virgin olive oil

2 corn tortillas (6 in. diameter)

1/4 avocado, sliced

1 oz thinly sliced cooked Chicken Breast (Boneless, Skinless)

1 leaf lettuce, cut into shreds

2 tsp Salsa (No-Salt-Added)

2 tsp minced fresh cilantro

Heat Extra Virgin Olive Oil over medium-high heat. Heat tortillas about a minute per side, until lightly browned. Remove tortillas from heat and lay flat.

On one tortilla, arrange avocado, chicken, lettuce, and salsa. Top with second tortilla.

🍎 Nutritional Facts x 1 Serving(s):

- Calories: 264
- Fat: 12 g
- Sat. Fat: 1 g
- Cholesterol: 24 mg
- Carbs: 27 g
- Sugars (Naturally-Occurring): 1 g
- Fiber: 6 g
- Protein: 12 g
- Sodium: 112 mg

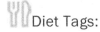 Diet Tags:

- 🌳 Gluten:
- 🥛 Dairy:
- 🌿 Acidic:
- 📦 Low Sodium: Yes
- 💚 Low Cholesterol: Yes
- ⬇ Low Carb:
- ⭕ Diabetics: Yes

Parmesan Popcorn

⌂ Makes: 1 🕐 Ready in: 4 min 🍴 Meal: Snack

Ingredients & Directions:

2 Tbsp Popcorn kernels.

1 Tbsp grated low-fat Parmesan cheese

2 tsp Extra Virgin Olive Oil

2 tsp water

2 pinches garlic powder

1 pinch sea salt

Pop the popcorn kernels

While popcorn is popping, whisk remaining ingredients in a bowl and microwave ten seconds.

Drizzle warm seasoning mixture over popped corn.

Nutritional Facts x 1 Serving(s):

- Calories: 130
- Fat: 2 g
- Sat. Fat: 0 g
- Cholesterol: 4 mg
- Carbs: 23 g
- Sugars (Naturally-Occurring): 1 g
- Fiber: 4 g
- Protein: 5 g
- Sodium: 125 mg

Diet Tags:

- 🌾 Gluten:
- 🥛 Dairy:
- Acidic: Yes
- Low Sodium: Yes
- Low Cholesterol: Yes
- Low Carb: Yes
- Diabetics: Yes

Chips and Guacamole

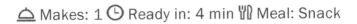

△ Makes: 1 🕐 Ready in: 4 min 🍴 Meal: Snack

Ingredients & Directions:

Nutritional Facts x 1 Serving(s):

1/3 avocado

2 Tbsp chopped tomato

1 Tbsp chopped onion

1 tsp fresh lime juice

1 pinch each garlic powder, chili powder, and sea salt.

Combine all ingredients and serve with ten tortilla chips.

- Calories: 130
- Fat: 2 g
- Sat. Fat: 0 g
- Cholesterol: 4 mg
- Carbs: 23 g
- Sugars (Naturally-Occurring): 1 g
- Fiber: 4 g
- Protein: 5 g
- Sodium: 125 mg

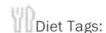Diet Tags:

- 🌳 Gluten:
- 🥛 Dairy:
- 🔥 Acidic: Yes
- 🧂 Low Sodium: Yes
- 💚 Low Cholesterol: Yes
- Low Carb: Yes
- ⭕ Diabetics: Yes

Bananas with Chocolate Fondue

🍽 Makes: 1 🕐 Ready in: 4 min 🍴 Meal: Snack

Ingredients & Directions:

3 Tbsp organic dark chocolate chips (at least 60% cacao)

1 sliced banana

Microwave chocolate chips until melted, ten seconds at a time to avoid scorching.

Microwave 3 Tbsp 60% organic dark chocolate chips 10 seconds at a time, stirring until melted.

Serve with banana slices.

Nutritional Facts x 1 Serving(s):

- Calories: 130
- Fat: 2 g
- Sat. Fat: 0 g
- Cholesterol: 4 mg
- Carbs: 23 g
- Sugars (Naturally-Occurring): 1 g
- Fiber: 4 g
- Protein: 5 g
- Sodium: 125 mg

Diet Tags:

- 🌾 Gluten:
- 🥛 Dairy:
- 🔥 Acidic:
- Low Sodium: Yes
- 💙 Low Cholesterol: Yes
- Low Carb: Yes
- Diabetics: Yes

Crackers with black olive tapenade

⌒ Makes: 1 ⏱ Ready in: 4 min 🍴 Meal: Snack

👨‍🍳 Ingredients & Directions:

8 Kalamata olives, pitted

1 tsp fresh lemon juice

½ tsp capers

½ tsp Extra Virgin Olive Oil

1 Pinch of pepper

Pulse all ingredients in blender until smooth.

Spread over whole grain crackers.

Nutritional Facts x 1 Serving(s):

- Calories: 130
- Fat: 2 g
- Sat. Fat: 0 g
- Cholesterol: 4 mg
- Carbs: 23 g
- Sugars (Naturally-Occurring): 1 g
- Fiber: 4 g
- Protein: 5 g
- Sodium: 125 mg

Diet Tags:

- 🌱 Gluten:
- 🥛 Dairy:
- 🔥 Acidic:
- 🧂 Low Sodium: Yes
- 💚 Low Cholesterol: Yes
- ↓ Low Carb: Yes
- ⭕ Diabetics: Yes

Peanut-Pretzel Trail Mix

Makes: 1 ⏰ Ready in: 4 min 🍴 Meal: Snack

Ingredients & Directions:

8 mini pretzel twists, broken

1 Tbsp each peanuts, pumpkin seeds, and dried currants.

Combine all ingredients and enjoy or store in a Ziploc bag to eat on the go.

Nutritional Facts x 1 Serving(s):

- Calories: 130
- Fat: 2 g
- Sat. Fat: 0 g
- Cholesterol: 4 mg
- Carbs: 23 g
- Sugars (Naturally-Occurring): 1 g
- Fiber: 4 g
- Protein: 5 g
- Sodium: 125 mg

Diet Tags:

- Gluten:
- Dairy:
- Acidic:
- Low Sodium: Yes
- Low Cholesterol: Yes
- Low Carb: Yes
- Diabetics: Yes

Curry Roasted Chickpeas

🍽 Makes: 1 🕐 Ready in: 4 min 🍴 Meal: Snack

Ingredients & Directions:

1 ½ tsp extra virgin olive oil

½ cup no salt added chickpeas, rinsed, drained, and dried

½ tsp curry powder

1 pinch each cumin, paprika, garlic powder, and sea salt.

Heat extra virgin olive oil over medium-high heat.

Add chickpeas

Cook 5-7 minutes stirring frequently.

Toss with seasoning mix.

🍎 Nutritional Facts x 1 Serving(s):

- Calories: 130
- Fat: 2 g
- Sat. Fat: 0 g
- Cholesterol: 4 mg
- Carbs: 23 g
- Sugars (Naturally-Occurring): 1 g
- Fiber: 4 g
- Protein: 5 g
- Sodium: 125 mg

Diet Tags:

- 🌳 Gluten:
- 🥛 Dairy:
- Acidic: Yes
- Low Sodium: Yes
- Low Cholesterol: Yes
- Low Carb: Yes
- Diabetics: Yes

Banana Berry Dream

 Makes: Serves 2. Each serving: 1 cup. ⏱ Ready in: 10 min 🍴 Meal: Snack

Ingredients & Directions:

1 banana, peeled and sliced

1 cup fresh strawberries, sliced

2 Tbsp Fat Free Vanilla Yogurt

2 Tbsp whole almonds or pecans

Directions:

Put half of the banana slices and strawberry slices in each of two dishes.

Top with yogurt and sprinkle with almonds.

Eat immediately.

Nutritional Facts x 1 Serving(s):

- Calories: 132
- Fat: 4 g
- Sat. Fat: 0 g
- Cholesterol: 0 mg
- Carbs: 21 g
- Sugars (Naturally-Occurring): 14 g
- Fiber: 4 g
- Protein: 3 g
- Sodium: 7 mg

Diet Tags:

- Gluten:
- Dairy:
- Acidic: Yes
- Low Sodium: Yes
- Low Cholesterol: Yes
- Low Carb: Yes
- Diabetics: Yes

Dinner

Broccoli Mushroom Omelet

✓

🔔 Makes: Serves 1 🕐 Ready in: 20 min 🍴 Meal: Dinner

Ingredients & Directions:

1/2 tsp Extra Virgin Olive Oil

1 cup sliced mushrooms

1 cup chopped broccoli

1/2 cup nonfat egg substitute

1/8 tsp black pepper

1/4 tsp oregano

Sauté mushrooms and broccoli in Extra Virgin Olive Oil until tender.

Add egg substitute.

Cover and cook over low heat until thoroughly cooked.

Sprinkle with pepper or oregano to taste.

Nutritional Facts x 1 Serving(s):

- Calories: 144
- Fat: 4 g
- Sat. Fat: 0 g
- Cholesterol: 0 mg
- Carbs: 10 g
- Sugars (Naturally-Occurring): 4 g
- Fiber: 3 g
- Protein: 17 g
- Sodium: 263 mg

Diet Tags:

- 🌳 Gluten:
- 🥛 Dairy:
- 🌿 Acidic: Yes
- 🧂 Low Sodium: Yes
- 💙 Low Cholesterol: Yes
- 🌾 Low Carb: Yes
- ⏲ Diabetics: Yes

Waldorf Salad

 Makes: Serves 4. 1 cup per serving. ⏱ Ready in: 5 min 🍴 Meal: Dinner

Ingredients & Directions:

3 apples, cored and diced

1 cup Fat Free Vanilla Yogurt

1/4 cup diced celery

1/4 cup Walnuts

green leafy lettuce for garnish

Combine all ingredients in a medium bowl.

Chill.

Serve cold on a bed of lettuce.

Sprinkle a pinch of ground cinnamon on top.

Nutritional Facts x 1 Serving(s):

- Calories: 149
- Fat: 5 g
- Sat. Fat: 0 g
- Cholesterol: 1 mg
- Carbs: 23 g
- Sugars (Naturally-Occurring): 12 g
- Fiber: 3 g
- Protein: 3 g
- Sodium: 43 mg

Diet Tags:

- 🌳 Gluten:
- 🥛 Dairy:
- Acidic: Yes
- Low Sodium: Yes
- Low Cholesterol: Yes
- Low Carb: Yes
- Diabetics: Yes

Southwestern Calico Corn

 Makes: 6 srv, 2/3 cup each ⏲ Ready in: 25 min 🍴 Meal: Dinner

Ingredients & Directions:

1 tbsp extra virgin olive oil

1 poblano pepper, diced and 1 small red bell pepper, diced

2 cups fresh corn kernels

1 tsp chili powder

1/2 tsp ground cumin

1/4 tsp salt

1 14-oz can hominy, rinsed

Heat Extra Virgin Olive Oil over medium-high heat. Add peppers and corn. Cook 3-5 minutes until just tender, stirring occasionally.

Stir in chili powder, cumin, and salt, continue cooking 30 seconds. Add hominy and cook another 2 minutes, stirring continuously.

Nutritional Facts x 1 Serving(s):

- Calories: 99
- Fat: 3 g
- Sat. Fat: 0 g
- Cholesterol: 0 mg
- Carbs: 16 g
- Sugars (Naturally-Occurring): 1 g
- Fiber: 3 g
- Protein: 2 g
- Sodium: 186 mg

Diet Tags:

- 🌳 Gluten:
- 🥛 Dairy:
- 🌊 Acidic: Yes
- Low Sodium: Yes
- ♥ Low Cholesterol: Yes
- Low Carb: Yes
- Diabetics: Yes

10 Minute Chili Soup

🛎 Makes: 4 - 1-1/4 cups ⏱ Ready in: 25 min 🍴 Meal: Dinner

👨‍🍳 Ingredients & Directions: ✓

1 tsp extra virgin olive oil

1 cup diced onions

1 cup diced carrots

1 can diced tomatoes

1 cup water

1 can kidney beans

1 tsp each chili powder and oregano

Sauté onions and carrots with oil in a preheated skillet three minutes, until golden and tender. Add remainder of ingredients and bring to a boil.

Reduce heat and simmer 4-5 minutes, until veggies are tender. Eat hot. Can be kept in a thermos or refrigerated and reheated.

🍎 Nutritional Facts x 1 Serving(s):

- Calories: 102
- Fat: 2 g
- Sat. Fat: 0 g
- Cholesterol: 0 mg
- Carbs: 17 g
- Sugars (Naturally-Occurring): 4 g
- Fiber: 6 g
- Protein: 4 g
- Sodium: 122 mg

🍴 Diet Tags:

- 🌱 Gluten:
- 🥛 Dairy:
- 🍋 Acidic:
- 🧂 Low Sodium: Yes
- ♥ Low Cholesterol: Yes
- ↓ Low Carb: Yes
- ○ Diabetics: Yes

Roasted Zucchini & Pesto

🍽 Makes: 4 srv, about 1 cup each ⏱ Ready in: 25 min 🍴 Meal: Dinner

👨‍🍳 Ingredients & Directions:

2 lbs zucchini, (about 4 medium), trimmed and cut into 1-in chunks

1 tbsp Extra Virgin Olive Oil

2 tbsp prepared pesto

Salt and black pepper to taste

Preheat baking sheet in 500°F oven.

While baking sheet is heating, toss zucchini with oil

Place zucchini in a single layer on baking sheet. Return to oven and roast 5-7 minutes.

Turn zucchini, continue roasting 7-9 minutes, until just tender. Toss roasted zucchini with pesto, salt, and pepper.

🍎 Nutritional Facts x 1 Serving(s):

- Calories: 111
- Fat: 7 g
- Sat. Fat: 2 g
- Cholesterol: 3 mg
- Carbs: 8 g
- Sugars (Naturally-Occurring): 0 g
- Fiber: 3 g
- Protein: 4 g
- Sodium: 119 mg

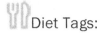 Diet Tags:

- 🌳 Gluten:
- 🥛 Dairy:
- 🔥 Acidic: Yes
- 🧂 Low Sodium: Yes
- 💛 Low Cholesterol: Yes
- 🍴 Low Carb: Yes
- ⭕ Diabetics: Yes

Cajun Sweet Potatoes

Makes: 4 ⏱ Ready in: 20 min 🍴 Meal: Dinner

Ingredients & Directions:

1 sliced sweet potato (raw)

2 tbsp Extra Virgin Olive Oil

2 tsp Chili powder

1/4 tsp Cajun Seasoning

Coat sweet potato slices with extra virgin olive oil. Sprinkle with chili powder and Cajun seasoning.

Grill over low heat, flipping occasionally, until it starts to get bubbly on the bottom.

Nutritional Facts x 1 Serving(s):

- Calories: 107
- Fat: 7 g
- Sat. Fat: 0 g
- Cholesterol: 0 mg
- Carbs: 10 g
- Sugars (Naturally-Occurring): 0 g
- Fiber: 1 g
- Protein: 1 g
- Sodium: 101 mg

Diet Tags:

- Gluten:
- Dairy:
- Acidic: Yes
- Low Sodium: Yes
- Low Cholesterol: Yes
- Low Carb: Yes
- Diabetics: Yes

Peach and Peanut Chicken Salad

🔔 Makes: srv: 6 srv 🕐 Ready in: 15 min 🍴 Meal: Dinner

👨‍🍳 Ingredients & Directions:

6 cups bite-size pcs salad greens

2 cups cut-up cooked chicken

2 cups sliced peaches

1 medium stalk celery, sliced (1/2 cup)

2 medium green onions, sliced (1/4 cup)

1/2 cup Light Raspberry Vinaigrette

1/2 cup honey-roasted peanuts, if desired

Toss all ingredient except peanuts in a large bowl.

Sprinkle peanuts on top.

Nutritional Facts x 1 Serving(s):

- Calories: 211
- Fat: 11 g
- Sat. Fat: 2 g
- Cholesterol: 40 mg
- Carbs: 14 g
- Sugars (Naturally-Occurring): g
- Fiber: 2 g
- Protein: 14 g
- Sodium: 90 mg

Diet Tags:

- 🌳 Gluten:
- 🥛 Dairy:
- 🍋 Acidic: Yes
- Low Sodium: Yes
- Low Cholesterol: Yes
- Low Carb: Yes
- Diabetics: Yes

Chicken Salad Lettuce Wraps

🛎 Makes: 8 - 2 wraps ⏱ Ready in: 10 min 🍴 Meal: Dinner

🧑‍🍳 Ingredients & Directions: ✓

1-1/2 cups cooked chicken breast

1 cup carrots, shredded

2 cups fresh spinach, chopped

1 cup fresh tomato, chopped

1 cup frozen corn, thawed

2 tsps garlic herb seasoning

1/4 cup reduced-fat mayonnaise

16 romaine lettuce leaves, washed

Mix all ingredients except lettuce leaves in a bowl.

Spread mixture on each lettuce leaf evenly. Roll lettuce leaf from one end. When you reach the middle, fold sides in and continue rolling.

🍎 Nutritional Facts x 1 Serving(s):

- Calories: 103
- Fat: 3 g
- Sat. Fat: 1 g
- Cholesterol: 24 mg
- Carbs: 9 g
- Sugars (Naturally-Occurring): 3 g
- Fiber: 2 g
- Protein: 10 g
- Sodium: 49 mg

🍴 Diet Tags:

- 🌳 Gluten:
- 🥛 Dairy:
- Acidic:
- Low Sodium: Yes
- 💚 Low Cholesterol: Yes
- Low Carb: Yes
- Diabetics: Yes

Zucchini and Peppers

 Ingredients & Directions:

1 zucchini

1 Green pepper

1 Red pepper

1 Banana pepper

1 Tomato

1 Onion

2 Tbsp Extra Virgin Olive Oil

Italian seasoning mix

Cut zucchini into 1 inch cubes.
Dice peppers, tomato, and onion.
Sauté all veggies in preheated pan
with extra virgin olive oil until
zucchini is tender. Sprinkle with
seasoning and stir.

 Nutritional Facts x 1 Serving(s):

- Calories: 131
- Fat: 7 g
- Sat. Fat: 0 g
- Cholesterol: 0 mg
- Carbs: 15 g
- Sugars (Naturally-Occurring): 1 g
- Fiber: 4 g
- Protein: 2 g
- Sodium: 13 mg

 Diet Tags:

- 🌳 Gluten:
- 🥛 Dairy:
- Acidic: Yes
- Low Sodium: Yes
- Low Cholesterol: Yes
- Low Carb: Yes
- Diabetics: Yes

Dessert

Strawberry Mango Dessert

🔔 Makes: 3 - 1/2 cup ⏰ Ready in: 5 min 🍴 Meal: Dessert

 Ingredients & Directions:

2 bananas

1/2 cup strawberries

1/2 mango, cut in strips

Freeze bananas and strawberries.

Process frozen bananas and strawberries in a food processor.

Garnish with mango.

 Nutritional Facts x 1 Serving(s):

- Calories: 125
- Fat: 1 g
- Sat. Fat: 0 g
- Cholesterol: 0 mg
- Carbs: 28 g
- Sugars (Naturally-Occurring): 19 g
- Fiber: 3 g
- Protein: 1 g
- Sodium: 2 mg

 Diet Tags:

- 🌳 Gluten:
- 🥛 Dairy:
- Acidic:
- Low Sodium: Yes
- Low Cholesterol: Yes
- Low Carb: Yes
- Diabetics: Yes

Orange Waldorf

🍲 Makes: Serves 4. Each serving: 3/4 cup. ⏰ Ready in: 10 min 🍴 Meal: Dessert

Ingredients & Directions:

3 oranges, diced

1 orange zest

1 apple, diced

1/4 cup Fat Free Vanilla Yogurt

2 Tbsp chopped walnuts

Stir all ingredients except walnuts together in a bowl.

Divide into four servings and top with walnuts.

Nutritional Facts x 1 Serving(s):

- Calories: 106
- Fat: 2 g
- Sat. Fat: 0 g
- Cholesterol: 0 mg
- Carbs: 19 g
- Sugars (Naturally-Occurring): 14 g
- Fiber: 3 g
- Protein: 3 g
- Sodium: 10 mg

🍴 Diet Tags:

- 🌳 Gluten:
- 🥛 Dairy:
- 🔥 Acidic: Yes
- Low Sodium: Yes
- 💚 Low Cholesterol: Yes
- Low Carb: Yes
- Diabetics: Yes

Paleo Coconut Chocolate Bars

🍽 Makes: 12 🕐 Ready in: 15 min 🍴 Meal: Dessert

👨‍🍳 Ingredients & Directions:

4 Tbsp. extra virgin olive oil

1/4 C. Unsweetened Cocoa Powder

1/2 C. Ground Nuts (Walnuts, Pecans or Almonds)

3/4 C. Shredded Coconut (unsweetened)

1 Tbsp. Honey

Chill a 9X9 baking pan. Combine dry ingredients together in a bowl. Stir in extra virgin olive oil and honey until well mixed.

Press into chilled baking pan and refrigerate at least 30 minutes. Cut into squares about ¾ to 1 inch.

Nutritional Facts x 1 Serving(s):

- Calories: 97
- Fat: 9 g
- Sat. Fat: 0 g
- Cholesterol: 0 mg
- Carbs: 3 g
- Sugars (Naturally-Occurring): 0 g
- Fiber: 1 g
- Protein: 1 g
- Sodium: 1 mg

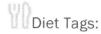 Diet Tags:

- 🌳 Gluten:
- 🥛 Dairy:
- Acidic: Yes
- Low Sodium: Yes
- Low Cholesterol: Yes
- Low Carb: Yes
- Diabetics: Yes

Hi-Phy Fruit Salad

 Makes: 4 - 3/4 cup Ready in: 5 min Meal: Dessert

Ingredients & Directions:

1 cup sliced canned peaches in juice

1 cup skinless red grapes, sliced in half

1 cup diced kiwi

1 cup sliced strawberries

1 tbsp chopped fresh mint

Combine all ingredients in medium bowl and chill.

Serve cold in small dessert glasses.

Nutritional Facts x 1 Serving(s):

- Calories: 121
- Fat: 1 g
- Sat. Fat: 0 g
- Cholesterol: 0 mg
- Carbs: 27 g
- Sugars (Naturally-Occurring): 20 g
- Fiber: 3 g
- Protein: 1 g
- Sodium: 6 mg

Diet Tags:

- Gluten:
- Dairy:
- Acidic:
- Low Sodium: Yes
- Low Cholesterol: Yes
- Low Carb: Yes
- Diabetics: Yes

Cool Six-Fruit Salad

🛎 Makes: 4 - 1 cup 🕐 Ready in: 10 min 🍴 Meal: Dessert

👨‍🍳 Ingredients & Directions:

1 cup strawberries, cut into halves

1 cup watermelon

1 sliced banana

1 peach or nectarine, cubed

1/2 cup grapes

1/2 cup orange juice

Gently stir all fruits together in a bowl.

Stir in orange juice.

Chill thoroughly, at least an hour.

Eat within 24 hours.

Nutritional Facts x 1 Serving(s):

- Calories: 100
- Fat: 0 g
- Sat. Fat: 0 g
- Cholesterol: 0 mg
- Carbs: 24 g
- Sugars (Naturally-Occurring): 17 g
- Fiber: 2 g
- Protein: 1 g
- Sodium: 2 mg

Diet Tags:

- 🌳 Gluten:
- 🥛 Dairy:
- Acidic:
- Low Sodium: Yes
- Low Cholesterol: Yes
- Low Carb: Yes
- Diabetics: Yes

Detox Waters

A good way to jumpstart your new lifestyle is to flush out some of the toxins that have accumulated as a result of years of unhealthy eating. The best way to detox is to flush your system with fresh, pure water. Problem is, water gets boring, that's why there are so many sodas and flavored waters on the market. To make a delicious detox water, put six cups of ice into a pitcher and add water to make 2 quarts. To the ice water, add any of the following recipes, stir and chill in the refrigerator for a couple of hours.

Grape Melon Medley

- 4 cups cantaloupe cut into small chunks
- 2 cups grape halves

Peach Pie

- 2 vanilla beans, gently crushed with a wooden spoon
- 6 peaches, pitted and sliced

Melon-Lime

- 3 limes, thinly sliced and muddled
- 4 cups honeydew, cut into small chunks

Sweet-Tart

- 2 cups chunk pineapple
- 1 cup cherries, pitted and cut in half
- 3 granny smith apples, cored and thinly sliced

Apples And Cinnamon

- 5 apples (your choice) cored and thinly sliced

- 5 whole cinnamon sticks

Plum Yum

- 6 fresh sage leaves, gently scrunched
- 10 plums, pitted and quartered
- 2 peaches, pitted and sliced

Cherries Jubilee

Muddle together:

- 2 cups cherries, pitted and halved
- 3 lemons, thinly sliced
- 2 vanilla beans

Fruit Cocktail

- 2 peaches, cored and sliced
- 2 pears, cored and sliced
- 2 cups grape halves
- 1 cup cherries, pitted and halved
- 1 cup pineapple chunks

Rosemary Refresher

- 4 sprigs rosemary, gently scrunched
- 6 cups watermelon chunks

Slightly Spicy

- 2 cucumbers, thinly sliced
- 2 jalapeño peppers, seeded and sliced

Citrus Sensation

Gently muddle:

- 2 lemons, thinly sliced
- 2 limes, thinly sliced,
- 2 grapefruits, thinly sliced
- 2 oranges, thinly sliced

Cucumber Quencher

- 6 sprigs mint, gently scrunched
- 2 cucumbers, thinly sliced,
- 4 limes, thinly sliced

Tropical Twist

- 2 cups pineapple chunks
- 2 cups fresh or frozen mango chunks
- 1 starfruit, thinly sliced

Sangria

Gently muddle:

- 4 cups grape halves
- 3 blood oranges, thinly sliced
- 2 apples, cored and thinly sliced

About the Authors

Enrico Forte, Bestselling Author, certified nutrition and wellness consultant, is an internationally renowned nutrition educator and culinary professional with an MBA master degree.

Valerie is a member of the Mediterranean Cuisine Academy (A.C.M.). We are nutrition educators, public speakers and members of the Alliance for Natural Health USA. We live in Catania, Italy with our family.

We're Italians, and the same principles in the book have worked for our families for centuries. This is the Mediterranean based dietary lifestyle after all! It can work for you too.

Closing Thoughts

Whew, we have covered just an enormous amount of information. You've just been handed a tremendous blueprint for living healthy. We've provided you with an in-depth look at how to build your healthy lifestyle.

The only thing left now is for you to take action.
We can tell you what to do and how to do it, but we can't make you do it.

That's up to you.

We will close out by reminding you of a wise saying we learned years ago that has monumentally changed our lives...

There are only two ways to get to the top of an oak tree.
One is to sit on an acorn and wait.
The other is to start climbing...
...See you at the top!

Health to you!
Enrico and Valerie Forte

Made in the USA
Columbia, SC
31 May 2018